IT'S NOT YOU, IT'S THE WORLD

IT'S NOT YOU, IT'S THE WORLD

A MENTAL HEALTH SURVIVAL GUIDE FOR US ALL

JOANNA CHEEK, MD

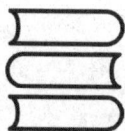

balance

New York Boston

Copyright © 2026 by Joanna Cheek
Foreword copyright © 2026 by Gabor Maté
Illustrations by Jackie Duys

Cover design by Terri Sirma. Cover image by Shutterstock.
Cover copyright © 2026 by Hachette Book Group, Inc.

Balance
Hachette Book Group
1290 Avenue of the Americas
New York, NY 10104
GCP-Balance.com
@GCPBalance

Originally published in 2026 by Collins, an imprint of Harper Collins Ltd., in Canada.
First U.S. Edition: February 2026

Balance is an imprint of Grand Central Publishing. The Balance name and logo are registered trademarks of Hachette Book Group, Inc.

The publisher is not responsible for websites (or their content) that are not owned by the publisher.

The Hachette Speakers Bureau provides a wide range of authors for speaking events. To find out more, go to hachettespeakersbureau.com or email HachetteSpeakers@hbgusa.com.

Balance books may be purchased in bulk for business, educational, or promotional use. For information, please contact your local bookseller or the Hachette Book Group Special Markets Department at special.markets@hbgusa.com.

Library of Congress Control Number: 2025948241

ISBNs: 978-0-306-83737-1 (hardcover), 978-0-306-83739-5 (ebook)

Printed in the United States of America

LSC-C

Printing 1, 2025

For our future

CONTENTS

FOREWORD

IN THIS FORWARD-LOOKING BOOK, PSYCHIATRIST JOANNA CHEEK PRESENTS AN ECO-logical view of human health and healing, bringing her skills as a journalist, meditation teacher, and psychotherapist to the task. By *ecological*, I mean far more than the usual physical environment that word usually denotes, for Dr. Cheek grounds her work and writing in the tradition-hallowed and scientifically unassailable view that all is one: the individual and the collective, the emotional and the physiological, the mind and the body, the culture and the family, the past and the present. Interwoven by multiple strands, each of these acts on the others, each manifests the others, each *is* the others. *Ecology* here includes both the external environment we inhabit but also the internal one that, if you will, inhabits us.

"Contemplate the nature of inter-connected co-arising during every moment . . ." said the Buddha 2,500 years ago. "The birth and death of any phenomena are connected to the birth and death of all other phenomena. The one contains the many and the many contains the one. Without the one, there cannot be the many. Without the many, there cannot be the one." If that unitary understanding of existence is not new, its incorporation into our culture's view of life and health, let alone into medical practice, is far from assured. Here, perhaps, Dr. Cheek is a tad more optimistic than reality may warrant. "We soon returned to our holistic views of the interconnected body and mind, with physicians now learning the bio-psycho-social-spiritual model of health," she says. *Some* physicians, I would say, here and there. Which is precisely what makes this book so essential, for our author makes a powerful case for that four-quadrant basis of wholeness, another word for which is *health*. All too often, there still yawns a vast chasm between what we know scientifically, or *should* know, on the one hand, and medical education and practice on the other. This has been called the *science-practice gap*. "Modern scientific medicine has taken a fundamentally materialist approach, and it is 'analytical,' meaning that it divides wholes into parts," so wrote the Canadian psychiatrist and author Norman Doidge. "It often proceeds by reducing complex phenomena to their more elementary chemical and physical components: viruses, genes, molecules . . ."

By contrast, Indigenous people worldwide, Joanna Cheek points out, have always held that health rests on a balance between our biological, psychic, social, and spiritual dynamics—the four segments of the North American "medicine wheel." Modern science has now more than amply demonstrated that natural unity. Among the merits of Dr. Cheek's work is to present in straightforward terms not only the evidentiary proof for that verity, but also insights, actions, and practices that can enable readers to incorporate its insights and wisdoms into their lives. Thus, this book more than instructs about healing; it makes healing into a practicable aim and endeavor.

In keeping with her fundamental message, the views, actions, and practices recommended by our author incorporate the intrapersonal, the interpersonal, the cultural and political, and even the historical. "The story of one life cannot be told separately from the story of other lives," the writer Susan Griffin has said. "Who are we? The question is not simple. What we call the self is part of a larger matrix of relationship and society. Had we been born to a different family, in a different time, to a different world, we would not be the same. All the lives that surround us are in us." Hence the pointed and poignant title of this book: *It's Not You*. Not you, that is, in isolation from all the influences that have helped to create and continue to shape who you are.

In this shame-based culture, many fear the stigma of having "problems," of being diagnosed with some "mental illness." On the other hand, modern psychiatry is all too prone to identify psychic and emotional distress as a biological flaw of the individual, often—it is claimed—rooted in genetics. *It's Not You, It's the World* fiercely challenges that perspective. It insists that we look at the wide-ranging circumstances that help create—if *help* is the right word in this highly noxious culture—who we believe we are, how we feel about ourselves, and how we experience our place in the world. And, yes, create even our biology and neurobiology. How, that is, social settings shape our internal environment. "We're still implicitly programmed from a lifetime of living in a hierarchical culture of dominance, division, and disposability," Dr. Cheek rightly asserts. "And we can be hard on ourselves and each other when our unconscious selves take the wheel, enacting old dynamics that drive us away from our ideals." That unconscious self, modulated by current social conditions and past trauma and its multigenerational transmission, too easily arrogates for itself the driver's seat in our lives; thus it is that we are literally "driven" into thought patterns, emotional states, and behaviors that do not serve and even undermine our natural needs and impulses for wholeness, for connection with others, and for belonging with and embracing the world.

With all that, nothing is further from Dr. Cheek's purpose in this work than having us see ourselves as the helpless and hapless victims of either past or present. Among her robust ABCs of restoring balance is agency, which she defines as engaging "in an activity that brings on a sense of mastery, autonomy, empowerment, or justice." Again, the personal is bound up with the social, for justice is, above all, a social concept. It's also deeply individual, for we must each find that mastery and resilience within ourselves. "While self-care is important, we need to care for both our embodied self and our collective self," Joanna Cheek teaches, "ensuring the health of all its connections and parts. If we stray too far into individualism, we deny our interdependence and collective self. And if we stray too far into collectivism, we may force conformity and intolerance of difference."

As much as the pathways to healing are to be forged in the mind, the recommendations in this book also take us into body. Dr. Cheek guides readers to anchor themselves in the physical reality of the moment. Attention to bodily sensations is key, for example, when we are triggered—noticing, as she says, when we are "on the dial of activation." Conscious breath and progressive muscle relaxation, with awareness, are among the many salutary practices she recommends.

Attending to ourselves—really noticing ourselves—is a necessary skill, all the more so since, as the author rightly says, not being fully seen as we are is one of our primal woundings, common from early childhood in a society that values people not for their authentic selves but for their attainments, accomplishments, and acquisitions—none of them sources of healthy self-esteem.

While a highly trained professional, Dr. Cheek does not cloak and armor herself in the white coat of academic expertise without sharing her own vulnerability. She has experienced burnout, anxiety, and depression. And shame. "As a queer woman, sudden waves of shame sometimes propel me to hide this part of myself when facing potentially homophobic groups of people that I predict will reject or harass me. My brain quickly and instinctively sets off its shame signal—'This part of you is bad'—as a shortcut to trigger the fast survival response of hiding the part that may be rejected." Our guide, in other words, has herself traversed the territory she leads us through. Who cannot relate? Who among us has not experienced shame? This is a guide we can trust.

"I've learned to hold compassion and empathy for everyone," Joanna Cheek tells us. In saying so, she has come to the position of nonjudgment upheld by spiritual masters of many faiths and disciplines ancient and current, and as reinforced by modern scientific insights into the social and interpersonal construction of both brain and personality. "Maybe extending compassion to a child whose dysregulation shows up as disruptive behavior is easier because we can clearly see the innocence of their stress responses," she says in one of the most potent passages in this book. "Can we offer the same compassion to ourselves and the adults around us whose so-called bad behavior we villainize? Rather than dehumanizing ourselves and others with blame and shame, can we see that our personal or historical trauma often steers our behaviors into ugly places simply to survive?"

The ultimate balm recommended in this fine work is compassion, for—as the physician and luminous writer Anton Chekhov contended—it is compassion "that moves us beyond numbness toward healing."

—GABOR MATÉ, MD
Internationally bestselling author of *The Myth of Normal: Trauma, Illness and Healing in a Toxic Culture*

IT'S NOT YOU,
IT'S THE WORLD

It is no measure of health to be well-
adjusted to a profoundly sick society.
—Jiddu Krishnamurti

AS A PSYCHIATRIST, I'M NOT SUPPOSED TO TALK ABOUT MYSELF. IT'S BEEN TRAINED OUT of me. So has reacting, desiring, hurting, hating, and really, being human. Freud Botoxed the hearts and faces of generations of us by preaching we be "blank screens" for you. We must be neutral so we don't interfere with your process. Who I am on the other side of the couch—with my muted heartbreaks and stifled rages—only obstructs my purpose: I'm here to help you.

It turns out that whittling us into well-trained robots doesn't create great doctors, nor does it prepare us to heal a diseased world. And ignoring and pushing down all the messy feelings inside awards us many health symptoms. (I've earned more diagnoses than degrees behind my name by now.) So, I'm relearning how to be human—and giving myself permission to frown, sob, giggle, and say no.

I wonder what's been trained out of you, too. Perhaps you've learned to push things down to cope in your environments, whether you needed to please, serve, protect, or survive. And maybe now you feel depressed, anxious, sick, or numb with all the things society keeps throwing at us to tranquilize that voice in our heads that screams, "Danger! This is not okay!"

Because our world isn't okay. If mental health symptoms are the canary, then the systems we inhabit are toxic. We need to feel distress when our world is endangered; because right now, it is. Our discomfort and despair and rage and fear are all the appropriate smoke alarms to a world on fire.

We're on the brink of climate disaster. Of spiraling conflict and division. Of ceasing to care for one another, supporting social systems that starve the majority to spoil a few; where the law's creators and courts are ruled by the highest bidders, while its enforcers kill and imprison those most oppressed. Of dehumanizing each other so much that we can't see supremacy as a terminal illness to society, where we can ignore, and even support, violence against anyone who appears not like us.

So, you're not broken or doing it wrong if you're stressed and struggling right now. We're designed to feel this distress: it's our alarm system to survive. And as our world is pushed to the brink of collapse, we need everyone's alarms to sound loud and clear to bring all our systems back into balance.

You might not be an instant fan of this idea, as I'm asking you to abandon the myth of self-improvement that promises if you alone could just act better or be better, then you'd avoid all the pain and flatline on happy. But self-help only bandages a cut without stopping the source of its bleeding.

Because these aren't isolated stresses harming our health: they're all connected. And their impact is not linear: the whole is greater than the sum of its parts. When one system collapses—whether our health, social systems, global relations, or ecosystems—the entire system collapses, not just within our own bodies and borders, but for the whole world. We're all in it together.

As each of us connects to every part of our planet through invisible links, "self-care" can't only focus on what's held within the boundaries of our bodies. To help ourselves, we must care for our collective: for all living beings and the ecosystems that support us all. An injury to any one part of our system is an injury to ourselves, just as a cell from the liver needs the health of the cells from the brain and heart to keep the whole body alive. As UN Secretary-General António Guterres explains, "Solidarity is self-interest. If we fail to grasp that fact, everyone loses."

So, maybe I've lost you already with no assurances of a quick fix. Or maybe you're noticing relief. Relief that you're not the only one who hurts, not the only one who lives in your head trying to ruminate a way out of it, who tries every escape hatch possible—for we're exceptionally creative at finding new ways to numb out, despite it only making things worse. Relief that we're all in this painful, uncertain mess together. Not that misery loves company, but that shame thrives in silence. Relief that it's not just you; it's the world.

Because this being human is hard. Life is suffering, taught the Buddha in his first Noble Truth, while Freud's greatest aspiration was to transform his patients' despair into common unhappiness.[1] Evolutionary psychologists explain how we've evolved to survive, not to be happy or calm.[2] You can think back to our ancestors, living thousands of years ago, staring off into the distance and thinking, *Is that a big, scary beast that can eat me or just a bush?* It wasn't the carefree ones who survived.[3] Those who managed to pass on their genes to the next generation were the stressed-out buzzkills who could imagine the worst from any situation.

And as a social species, we're designed for connection, depending on group membership to survive. So, fears of separation and rejection are also favored to keep us alive.

But anxiety, grief, and rejection feel painful in the same way as a splitting headache, because emotional and physical pain share the same neural pathways in the brain. It's no wonder we're trained to avoid this distress. We habitually numb out with food, alcohol, and drugs, or we distract with work, screens, and overscheduling. We consume ourselves with fixing everyone else's problems instead of feeling our own, or we get lost in thoughts, obsessing about the future and past rather than noticing what's right here. We blame everyone around us instead of experiencing the vulnerable emotions underneath—at least rage feels powerful.

Yet even our most painful feelings serve important functions. The biggest obstacle to healing our world isn't heated opposition but apathy. It's not the hard deniers—those screaming in all caps that the science of climate change is a hoax—who stop us from saving ourselves, warns climate activist Naomi Klein. It's the soft deniers, "The rest of us who know it's real but act like it's not, who keep forgetting, in a myriad of ways, both large and small."[4]

Because we need to be distressed when our world is endangered. "There are some things in our social system that I'm proud to be maladjusted to, and I call upon you to be maladjusted too," urged Dr. Martin Luther King Jr. as he commended the victory of fifty thousand appropriately distressed Black Americans in Alabama who boycotted the racial segregation of buses in 1956. "The salvation of our world lies in the hands of the maladjusted," he affirmed.

OUR DISTRESS ISN'T THE PROBLEM

Yet we often learn to blame or shame ourselves when we hurt. Maybe it's more comfortable than sitting with the heavy reality that the world around us is sick in overwhelmingly complex ways. If it's only us, then it's easier to fix. I wish I could tell you to just breathe and think happy thoughts and you'll be magically cured of this pain, that everything will be fine. But it's not just you that's the problem.

Our distress alarms blare because we're exposed, relentlessly, to the imbalances in our complex systems, which constantly assault us with toxic stress. For many of us, the stress is social. Maybe you feel alone, unseen, or hurt by others. Or maybe you're triggered by memories of injustice, abuse, and heartbreak, or haunted by the old taunts of past bullies. Or perhaps your caregivers' incapacity to meet your needs as a child now corrupts your current relationships.

Maybe your stress is historical, that your ancestors were dehumanized, colonized, or discriminated against for their class, culture, or color of skin. Or intergenerational, that your relatives passed down their adaptations to their own traumas from war, oppression, or abuse. Or the stress is political, with daily exposures to supremacy, inequities, and conflict constantly setting off your alarms.

The stress may be biological, from exposures to infections, toxins, or diseases that threaten your body. Or environmental, because you're affected by wildfires, pollution, or the fear of bringing children into an unsustainable world. Maybe your stress is spiritual, that you feel disconnected from your higher power, purpose, or sense of connection to our larger web of life. Too often, our mental health struggles come from all of these entangled stressors, all of the time.

So, before we learn strategies to soothe our symptoms, we must listen closely to what they're signaling. Our distress is not the problem. It alerts us to problems, that dear friend who tells us the truths we need to hear, rather than the reassurances we desire. It signals that the dynamic systems we live in—whether they be our bodies, social systems, or ecosystems—need attention and care to bring them back to balance. Silencing these alarms doesn't make them go away; it just forces them to scream louder.

IT MAKES SENSE YOU HURT

While it makes sense that we're struggling right now, we keep hearing messages that we shouldn't feel this way.

Has anyone ever responded to your distress with any of the following statements?

"You're overreacting or too sensitive."
"You should be happy. Think of all the people living in a war zone."

"We're not racist/sexist/ableist/classist/homophobic."

"Why don't you just think positively?"

"Just let it go."

How do those statements land for you?

Anyone who throws me a "Just relax" will transform my typically pleasing grin into the glare of a tween whose parents just took away her screens. Marsha Linehan, the creator of dialectical behavior therapy (DBT), learned a hard lesson by doing just that. As she began counseling as a new clinician, she realized that the more she threw advice at her clients, the worse they felt.[5]

What she missed was validating and accepting their pain—simply communicating, "Ouch. It makes sense that you hurt"—which is now the foundation of DBT. We invalidate our emotions when we reject our inner experiences or oversimplify the problems that they signal. Instead, we need to both acknowledge the hurt that's present and understand how hard the situation really is. Validating tells our brains that our distress signals are heard so they no longer need to keep sounding. It's an essential step in coping with painful experiences, whether approaching our own or when supporting others.

So, your distress makes sense and I'm not going to oversimplify the situation: healing the entangled mess of a failing world is a huge task.

You might be sensing by now that I have my share of three-in-the-morning panic spirals, worrying if I'm doing enough—if we're collectively doing enough—to bring our systems into balance. Yet our distress gives us power: we can't solve the problems that we don't see.

And I alone can't see everything, nor do I have all the answers. The limited lens of one person could never understand all the complexities of our interconnected systems, in both sickness and health. Nor am I neutral. We can't deny the immeasurable influences that shape how each of us interacts with the world, from our unique biology to our ever-changing adaptations to our histories, environments, cultures, and intersecting social positions of power and privilege.

Recognizing our biases and knowledge gaps is murky at best, and more like trying to find a lost contact lens without wearing our glasses. So, as a white, cisgendered, queer, able-bodied Canadian settler residing on the stolen Indigenous homelands of the ləkʷəŋən-speaking peoples of the Songhees and Esquimalt Nations, I can't pretend to be an objective expert on your health, or on the world that's making us sick—I'm distinctly impacted by it, too.

It might feel like a plot twist, then, to mention that I'm a perky optimist, full of hope for the future. Because no one person needs to know or solve it all. But each of us can help with one of the world's problems. And if we come together with all our unique skills and perspectives, we could solve most of them. "We are the guides we most need," teaches activist Mia Birdsong, as she pushes for social change by leveraging the "brilliance of everyday people."

Yet as our world becomes increasingly sick, our alarms won't stop sounding, immobilizing so many of us into denial or despair. So, my contribution is this mental health survival guide. I'll share a wide assortment of tools to help us understand and work with the alarms that our ailing systems keep signaling. Then we can see and solve our shared problems that keep setting them off.

As we're all so beautifully diverse in our histories, biologies, social contexts, and needs, I invite you each to play with these offerings to explore what's most helpful for you: adapt some, discard others, and take what you need. Throughout the book, I'll also provide real-life examples that may echo your own painful experiences. Please approach this content gently by noticing its impact on your body, and then choose to dose, delay, or disregard any sections that may feel too overwhelming for you in each moment. You are the expert of your own needs and we each require unique paths to healing.

COLLECTIVE HEALING

> Without inner change, there can be no outer change,
> without collective change, no change matters.
> —Rev. angel Kyodo williams

We need to care for our world as if our lives depend on it. Because collective-care is self-preservation. And together, we can tend to both.

While we may doubt our capacity to rise to this moment, so many of our heroes "had ordinary lives, but life pulled the extraordinary out of them," says Susan Abulhawa in *Against the Loveless World*. The pandemic taught us how rapidly we could unite across the globe to shift our social structures and innovate in ways that we could never before fathom. Let's use the gravity of our current crises to come together to pivot yet again.

As Lilla Watson declared as she spoke at the 1985 UN Decade for Women Conference: "If you have come here to help me, you are wasting your time. But if you have come because your liberation is bound up with mine, then let us work together."

IT'S NOT
YOU,
IT'S THE
WORLD

ONE

WE'VE EVOLVED TO SURVIVE, AND BE MISERABLE

I was fortunate to find myself struggling with severe depression.
Of course, back then, it wasn't a blessing. It was a pain in the
ass. I say it's a blessing now because for me, in my life, it's
always been great moments of struggle and great moments of
suffering that have lit the fire under me to change. I started
asking, "Okay, but what else? What am I missing?"
—LAMA ROD OWENS

———————

PEOPLE COME TO SEE ME FOR HELP WITH THEIR DEPRESSION, ANXIETY, EATING DISOR-
ders, addictions, or any other label that fails to adequately describe
why we hurt. These diagnoses take on a life of their own, as we try to
treat the "depression" or "anxiety" instead of addressing the problems
that these symptoms are signaling. But what if the mixture of mental
health struggles we face aren't the primary problem? What if these
symptoms started as signals to help us see or solve the problems in our
environments?

One in two of us will be diagnosed with a mental health condition by the age of forty, with one in five experiencing an active episode each year.[1] It's hard to view all of our mental health challenges
as disordered if so many of us are experiencing them. Perhaps it's not

that something's gone wrong in our bodies and minds, but that something's gone right. Maybe these symptoms are brilliant alarms and adaptions to survive a disordered world.

"The key view in evolutionary theory is that if we find behaviors that we do not like or cause suffering to self or others, we should not automatically assume that something has gone wrong 'in the machine,'" says Paul Gilbert, a professor at the University of Derby, who's researched evolutionary psychology for over thirty-five years.[2] Rather, he asks, "In what social contexts are these behaviors prevalent? What functions are they serving?"

Remember how we've evolved to survive, and not to be happy or calm? Low mood, anger, shame, anxiety, envy, guilt, and grief are all helpful signals to meet the challenges of our specific environments. Having sensitive protective functions that sound alarms or short-circuit when we're threatened isn't a design flaw. It's a design success.

Psychobiologist Jaak Panksepp spent a lifetime studying the neuroscience of emotions to show how we all have seven distinct emotional networks organized within the lower subcortical parts of our brains: separation distress (grief/panic), fear, rage, seeking, lust, care, and play.[3] "They are ancestral tools for living," Panksepp explained, which help us meet our needs, protect against threats, and return our systems to balance. Throughout our lives, we refine these primary emotional circuits with unconscious learning (known as *conditioning*) from our environments, adjusting the sensitivity of each network to meet the specific needs of our unique settings. Then, we consciously interpret our feelings in the higher parts of our thinking brain to shape our emotional experiences even further.

If it sounds complicated, it is. Even the people who study emotions rarely agree on a specific number of emotions or how we experience them, especially when our cultural context impacts how we learn and think about emotions. In later chapters, we'll explore how most of our struggles with emotions are not straightforward responses to the present situation. Instead, our messy emotional reactions, with their associated thinking biases and impulses to act, arise as adaptations to a lifetime of experiences.

But let's start with the basics of this brilliant evolutionary alarm system to understand why it's so good to feel so bad.

IT'S BETTER TO BE SAFE THAN SORRY

Inside a single-use life, there are no second chances.

—OCEAN VUONG

Psychiatrist Randolph Nesse, founding director of the Center for Evolution and Medicine at Arizona State University, began his career directing an anxiety disorders clinic. He found himself asking why we have panic attacks in situations that seem safe.[4] But then he came across the smoke detector theory. "I started realizing that it's essential for alarms to go off, even if there's just a chance of danger. When the threat is uncertain, false alarms are worth it," Nesse says.

When the probability of harm in our environment is greater than the cost of fear, it's helpful to experience anxiety, even if it means having an unnecessary panic attack in a crowded subway. "I finally understood that the system is set to have many, many normal false alarms," says Nesse. We adapt to the challenges of our environments by changing the sensitivity of our alarms to match the perceived threats around us. If a lot of danger is lurking outside, our survival depends on sounding alarms every time we leave the house so we're primed to hypervigilance and prepared to protect ourselves.

Social activist and Buddhist minister Lama Rod Owens describes how fear helps him survive the dangers of living as a Black man amid the ongoing racial violence in the US in *Love and Rage: The Path of Liberation Through Anger:*

When Trayvon Martin was murdered, I stopped wearing black hoodies. When Tamir Rice was murdered, I thought about how to give up my hands so I wouldn't be mistaken for holding on to anything. When Renisha McBride was murdered, I vowed never to knock on any stranger's door again. When Sandra Bland and Walter Scott were murdered, I became hypervigilant about following every fucking driving law. When Eric Garner was choked to death, I realized that we all had been choking. After Akai Gurley was killed, I tried to figure out how to always make noise so no one would ever be surprised by me. After Freddie Gray was murdered, I thought there was surely a way not to be Black any longer. After Charles Kinsey was shot, I began questioning why would I help anyone if the cops would simply show up and shoot me anyway.[5]

As Owens describes, fear is a life-saving signal to help us survive potential threats that resemble those we or others have encountered before. It protects us in dangerous environments. But it's not only our own experiences that set our alarm's sensitivity; we adapt to the threats that our ancestors faced, too.

INTERGENERATIONAL WISDOM

> If we carry intergenerational trauma, then we
> also carry intergenerational wisdom.
> —Kazu Haga

The pandemic punted many of us into a foreign world where our past adaptations failed. Suddenly, even grocery shopping felt like a game of Pac-Man, as we outran the ghosts of former friends who transformed into scary monsters the moment they got within arm's reach.

I felt the collective anxiety grow all around me. Except for one place: my clinic. People I'd been seeing for years for severe and persistent post-traumatic stress disorder, obsessive-compulsive disorder, complex trauma, addictions, chronic self-harm, suicidality, depression, and anxiety disorders, who'd spent their lives hearing from society that they were too sensitive or overreacting, suddenly thrived.

I should know, because I was one of them.

After years of treatment for my many symptoms of anxiety, it turned out that all I needed to feel better was to be dropped into a deadly pandemic—that is, an environment that matched the setting of my super-reactive smoke detector.

I rocked Covid. At least at the start. I worked long hours of over-time leading a mental health response to support our frontline work-ers, creating and presenting stress first-aid workshops to groups across my province, all while developing the daily ritual of clearing a smooth path of open doors from outside the house into the shower for my co-parent, a doctor working on the COVID-19 wards, who stripped off every piece of contaminated clothing in the backyard shed.

It all seemed oddly calm and normal. Yes, we had a high risk of dying, I thought at the time, but I felt deeply at peace with it. Finally, the rest of the world validated my anxiety. Finally, everyone else could see what I'd been preparing for my entire life, that the world was a terrifying place.

I've always been anxious. My kids came screaming out of the womb anxious. As I look through the generations on both sides of my family, I see different shades of anxiety—or attempts to obliterate it with addictions or depression. As I trace back one side of my family, my great-grandmother received a lobotomy in an attempt to treat her unremitting depression, followed by mental health struggles in the generations that followed. On the other side, my Ukrainian great-grandmother fled Russia with her seven children to escape the Tsar's violence and discrimination, only to then leave my great-grandfather when he gambled away their new life in attempts to numb the grief of losing their old one. History repeated itself when her daughter, my grandma, lost my grandpa to addiction once again.

I lived with this grandma, who raised me on a steady diet of cabbage rolls, pickled herring, and interminable grief, after she also lost her only daughter to an autoimmune disease. We didn't talk much about our family history. But I trust there must have been good reasons for our smoke alarms to be set this way. The defining feature of trauma is that it goes unspoken; it's not expressed in words as much as burned into our bodies.

Instead, the stories I learned as a kid were of my grandma's resilience. How she left her humble family farm at sixteen to travel alone to New York to train as a hairstylist. How she returned to Canada in her twenties to start her own salon, which thrived during the Great Depression and Second World War, all while rowing her boat to work every day from her home on a tiny island. How she slept with such sturdiness each night, as she let me cuddle right up to the heat of her cracked skin, that her bed felt like my only safe haven in a scary world. How she lived off fried sausages and cigarettes, and yet, as her friends and family died all around her, there she was, the last woman standing, still tap dancing in our kitchen in her eighties. Give my grandmother hardship, and she flourished.

THE TRANSMISSION OF TRAUMATIC STRESS BETWEEN GENERATIONS

We are not makers of history. We are made by history.
—MARTIN LUTHER KING JR.

———

Why is life so full of suffering? Because emotional responses benefit our genes, not us, Nesse explains.[6] In 1859, biologist Charles Darwin first described how natural selection shapes organisms to behave in ways that maximize their reproductive success. While diseases themselves are not adaptations, traits that make us more vulnerable to disease do make evolutionary sense if they help us survive long enough to reproduce.

Remember how the most anxious and insecure of us won the game of natural selection? If our environments were particularly hostile, then these anxious traits would be even more likely to be selected and passed on to the next generations through our genes, despite the burden of mental health symptoms that they carried.

Our ancestors passed down their adaptations to threats from their own environments. If our parents were exposed to discrimination, war, poverty, violence, colonialism, abuse, or anything that created a lack of safety and security, then we are lucky to come out of the womb screaming and ready to fight such hostile environments. We don't need to learn the hard way from our own experiences, which could be fatal. Instead, our marvelous system can pass on adaptations through the generations by altering the sensitivity of our threat and reward networks.

Lama Rod Owens illustrates how his body also carries the memories of generations of his ancestors facing the trauma and tragedy of white supremacy:

> I am the little girl at the bottom of the ocean. I am the teenage
> boy in the belly of the ship. I am the young girl displayed on the
> auction block. I am the grandmother singing songs about someone
> else's god. I am the father in the fields with tobacco and cotton.
> I am the woman raped by my master. I am the baby born from
> the violence. I am the husband forced to watch. I am the same
> husband, who will be raped by his master's wife. I am the boy
> raped by the slave master. I am the mother who will never see her
> children again. I am the grandfather who will never know he was
> a grandfather. I am the one buried in an unmarked grave. I am the
> one hunting me.

As Owens shows us, this adaptive capacity comes at a cost, as these intergenerational adaptations also carry the heavy burden of grief, anger, or anxiety that's inherited alongside them. Psychiatrist

Vivian Rakoff, former chair of the Department of Psychiatry at the University of Toronto, first published a paper in 1966 describing how trauma is observed in the children of those exposed to it, despite not experiencing the trauma themselves. "The parents are not broken conspicuously," wrote Rakoff of his patients who were the children of Holocaust survivors. "Yet their children, all of whom were born after the Holocaust, display severe psychiatric symptomatology. It would almost be easier to believe that they, rather than their parents, had suffered the corrupting, searing hell."[7]

Rakoff's paper received a lot of pushback. Among its biggest criticisms was how acknowledging intergenerational trauma could be stigmatizing to survivors' descendants, as it changes the narrative from resilience to one of being broken, says Rachel Yehuda, psychiatrist and director of the Traumatic Stress Studies Division at the Icahn School of Medicine at Mount Sinai in New York.[8] But what if these changes observed in future generations weren't dysfunctional but highly adaptive?

Yehuda is known around the world as a leading expert in traumatic stress, penning over five hundred published papers, chapters, and books on the topic. She explains how a variety of mechanisms transmit traumatic stress to our children: through epigenetics, in utero, and behaviorally.[9] Epigenetics focuses on how we turn on or off our genes—without changing our actual DNA code itself—by adding or removing signals to our DNA in response to our environments. While studying generations of people is difficult, many animal studies show how trauma-induced epigenetic changes in DNA can be passed through the generations. Human studies are still in their infancy but suggest the same conclusion.

"The implications of these findings may seem dire, suggesting that parental trauma predisposes offspring to be vulnerable to mental health conditions," Yehuda explains.[10] "But some evidence suggests that the epigenetic response may serve as an adaptation that might help the children of traumatized parents cope with similar adversities." When children's alarms are fine-tuned to meet the specific needs of the hostile environments that their parents have already adapted to, they are more likely to survive these threats.

We also pick up cues in the womb to help us survive. If parents are living in dangerous environments, their stress system adapts by becoming more sensitive. Their babies will then take cues from being exposed to stress hormones in utero and sensitize their own alarm systems to better detect potential dangers.[11] In this way, the babies arrive in what they predict to be a hostile environment ready to cope with its threats. They experience more false alarms, but since the odds of danger are probably high, the increased anxiety is worth it.

Children then adapt the sensitivity of alarms to their caregiver's capacity to connect with them.[12] If their caregivers seem preoccupied with safety or paying rent, their children will adapt their own alarms to be more anxious or avoidant to help them survive this tougher world. But if caregivers live in safe and supportive environments that allow them to be more calm and attentive, and thus able to respond to their kin in a more secure way, then their children's stress response doesn't have to be set so high, and they, too, assume the privilege of being less reactive to stress.

Feeling low levels of anxiety is not a personal triumph; it's a privilege. It simply means that both you and your ancestors had the luck of living in secure environments, bestowed with both physical and emotional safety.

THE GIFTS OF A LOW MOOD

We have seasons when we flourish and seasons when the leaves fall
from us, revealing our bare bones. Given time, they grow again.
—KATHERINE MAY

Our moods can crash when we face loss, sickness, relationship problems, isolation, the realities of systemic inequities, the myriad of ways we can burn out, and even with more neutral events like life transitions and the long, dark days of winter. But low mood is also a helpful adaptation to meet our needs.

Imagine you are fishing and catching plenty of trout, Randolph Nesse teaches. We're designed to feel upbeat to motivate us to keep going in this highly productive situation. But then, as the fish start to dwindle, we begin to feel down. This is the early sign that the rewards are no longer worth the risk of all the potential lions and tigers and bears that may eat us if we keep fishing in the same spot. Our frustrated seeking system motivates us to risk the uncertain journey of giving up on a lake to find a more rewarding fishing spot somewhere else.

If we keep fishing and still nothing, our body's seeking system goes into hibernation mode as the perceived risk of harm in our environments outweighs the potential rewards, says Nesse. Our low-mood alarm signals to us to go back to the safety of our caves, cuddle under the covers, and wait until the fish come back. A low mood is not a personal failure or weakness; it's a sign that our environment's rewards don't outweigh the risks of leaving our caves. Our seeking systems hibernate to help us conserve energy during the gray seasons of life.

At the same time, our evolutionary alarms aren't that fine-tuned, only sensing immediate rewards, not the long-term picture. When we transition through new journeys in life—even when we're moving in a desired direction—our alarms may sense an immediate state of reduced reward in relation to the increased threats from risk and uncertainty. It takes time to find and harvest new rewards. For this reason, life transitions, both wanted and unwanted, often bring on a low mood. It's like we're a hermit crab that's outgrown its shell. We need to leave our shell to find one that fits better, but to do so, we must lose the rewards of our old shell until we finally find and reap the benefits of the bigger shell in the future.

The quiet ache of my own persistent low mood pushed me to trade in the comfort and care of my low-conflict marriage to my kind ex-husband to come out as queer. The distress of low mood made the consequences of not acting more painful than the disruptive journey of change. While this transition initially brought on a lot of distress, my bouts of low mood eventually lifted as I began feeling the rewards of living authentically, aligned with my values.

So, when our low-mood signals arise with the pull of unhappiness or hibernation, rather than immediately trying to rid ourselves of the discomfort, we can get curious about the message it's trying to communicate. Does our current environment offer more risks than rewards? Is this situation one we can wait out until the next season brings back the fish, such as during the winter or a bout of illness? Or do we need to change our approach to create more rewards, whether trying out new settings, relationships, pursuits, or ways of living?

And what if the entire world's environment is high risk and low reward? As we face runaway inequities, global conflict, and the collapse of our climate, the warning signals of low mood can push us all to see the problems so we can fix them. What collective actions do we need to ensure our entire planet is safe and sustainable, so that its harms don't forever outweigh its rewards?

GRATITUDE FOR OUR GRIEF

As we evolved into humans by growing big, impressive brains, we faced quite a design flaw: How would we get these huge baby heads out of their mothers' tiny pelvises? We adapted to this problem by giving birth to our offspring early, when they're much less developed than that of other species, leaving our young dependent on caregivers to survive until they're mature enough to function on their own. As a social species, this interdependence on others persists across our lifespans, as we continue to need connection and group membership to survive. For this reason, one of the biggest alarm systems in our brains is the attachment alarm that alerts us to threats to our bonding to others with pronounced feelings of separation distress.

Our attachment alarms ring with separation distress when our loved ones are unavailable or inconsistent, such as when they're preoccupied with other people or activities instead of attending to our relationship or needs. These alarms sound as jealousy when we sense that the person we love or depend on may be taken from us. At its loudest, it expresses heartbreak and grief, when we've completely lost an important relationship.

While loss can drive us to retreat into our cave with low mood, because we no longer have access to the rewards of what we've lost, it can also bring on an intense feeling of grief or panic, which motivates us to seek out supports and restore the sense of attachment and security that we've lost. I remember when a past partner broke up with me, every muscle of my body folded into the heavy feeling of heartbreak. As she watched my body crumble right before her, I could sense her discomfort grow, pushing her to apologize for her role in my pain.

"Yes, I'm hit with grief right now," I told her, "and it's not bad to feel this way. It's telling me that this relationship matters and being in a partnership like this is important to me." When I used my grief alarm to show me what's important, I instantly felt gratitude for having had this connection in my life and hoped I could find it again. Whenever I felt a wave of grief come up as I healed, rather than isolating, which only made me feel worse, I tried to reestablish my sense of bonding to others, connecting more with friends and then dating again, as it kept reminding me how much love matters. The attachment alarm hurt—a hell of a lot—but it moved me to quickly regain what I had lost and to express gratitude for what I have. Grief is a compass to our heart, allowing us to see what's important, so we can rebuild it.

Many of us are feeling a similar grief for our larger world as humans keep destroying the health of our ecosystems and societies. This grief alarm, while deeply painful, also alerts us to our deep connection to these living systems. We're grieving because we all need our world's health to survive. And just like with heartbreak, it can motivate us to fight to regain what we've lost: a just, caring, and sustainable world.

"Only we, the heartbroken, can truly battle and long for a world where no-one ever feels like this again," argues Gargi Bhattacharyya, a professor of sociology at the University of East London. "Who can imagine another world unless they already have been broken apart by the world we are in."

SHAME: IT'S NOT YOU, IT'S THEM

I am not trapped in the wrong body; I am trapped in a
world that makes very little space for bodies like mine.
—IVAN COYOTE

For years, I taught that all the emotions have important roles, except shame. Shame was the screwup of the family, the one we wished could just act like its perfect sibling, guilt, who was polite and cleaned up after all its messes.

The guilt alarm signals the helpful message, *I did something bad*, and pushes us to repair the situation, while shame sends the short warning, *I am bad*, urging us to hide and deny the perceived flaw. While the guilt signal sends many false alarms, just like all the others, we often see it as the golden child because it motivates us to be accountable and repair the fracture, while shame pushes us to conceal our perceived problem (or shift the blame to others). For this reason, we teach caregivers to discipline their children with, "I love you, and not this behavior," to encourage accountability and self-compassion.

But guilt doesn't beat out shame in all situations. Sometimes, we must hide even the most beautiful parts of ourselves. "To be gorgeous, you must first be seen, but to be seen allows you to be hunted," writes Ocean Vuong in my favorite book, *On Earth We're Briefly Gorgeous*. When we sense the threat of being shunned by others if we were to fully show up, our survival instincts push us to hide the parts of ourselves that others may reject. The distress of this signal pushes us to find a safer community, or hide parts of ourselves if we're stuck needing to appease groups that would reject this part of us.

"To understand vulnerability, one has to fully grasp the concept of psychological safety"—the belief that one will not be punished, humiliated, or rejected for showing one's authentic self, explains behavioral scientist Carey Yazeed, author of *Everyday Struggle: How Toxic Workspaces Impact Black Women*.[13] She warns that the "courage culture" of expressing our vulnerability that's celebrated by people who rest safely in social positions of power and privilege can be dangerous for more marginalized people. Instead, when exploring the benefits of vulnerability, Yazeed teaches that we must first learn how to do it safely within the world that we live in—sharing our vulnerability only to those who are safe enough to receive it.

As with fear, the alarm of shame can signal unsafe situations. When we enter environments where we don't feel psychological safety, our shame alarms ring loudly, warning us to pause and assess our risk of rejection and ridicule if we were to show our authentic selves. And also as with fear, we experience many false alarms, especially if our shame signals learned early on to be more sensitive as an adaptation to experiences of past harm, criticism, or rejection from others, whether personally or intergenerationally.

As a queer woman, sudden waves of shame sometimes propel me to hide this part of myself when facing potentially homophobic groups of people that I predict will reject or harass me. My brain quickly and instinctively sets off its shame signal—*This part of you is bad*—as a shortcut to trigger the fast survival response of hiding the part that may be rejected. My brain doesn't have time to process the longer story of how the shame is really signaling to me how potentially rejecting this community is—or has been in the past—and has nothing to do with my own worthiness as an individual. My shame alarm tells me that it's safer to hide this gorgeous part of myself because these people can't be trusted with it.

Australian comedian Hannah Gadsby, who identifies as gay and gender nonbinary, spoke about being raised in Tasmania, where same-sex love was a crime until 1997, in their famous show *Nanette*. "Seventy percent of the people who raised me, who loved me, who I trusted, believed that homosexuality was a sin, that homosexuals were heinous, subhuman, pedophiles. Seventy percent!" Gadsby said. "And by the time I identified as being gay, it was too late, I was already homophobic. And you do not get to just flip a switch on that."

Gadsby's mother told them, "The thing I regret is that I raised you as if you were straight. I didn't know any different. I'm so sorry. I knew well before you did, that your life was going to be so hard. I knew that, and I wanted, more than anything in the world, for that not to be the case. And now I know that I made it worse. I made it worse because I wanted you to change, because I knew that the world wouldn't."

Gadsby now refuses to use self-deprecating humor in their comedy shows to relieve the tension created in their audience when speaking about being abused for who they are. They now see the tension they feel, the deep shame of rejection from both strangers and those they loved—the "damage done to me [that] is real and debilitating"—as no longer theirs to relieve. They're giving it back to its rightful owner, the dominant society that created it. "This tension is yours. I am not helping you anymore," Gadsby concludes. "You need to learn what this feels like, because this tension is what 'not-normals' carry inside of them all of the time. It is dangerous to be different."

Shame is an essential—albeit excruciating—signal to alert us to situations where our belonging or safety would be at risk if we were to show up fully as we truly are. We need it to survive. But we also need to remember that shame is a fast-acting warning—and one with many false alarms learned from the past—that screams something's bad about us so we will react quickly enough to hide and survive in a group that is primed to reject us. We must honor the slower, more complete story of shame. It's not actually you that's the problem; it's those who reject you.

IF YOU'RE NOT ANGRY, YOU'RE NOT PAYING ATTENTION

Right now, we have a lot to be angry about. Anger is a necessary response to fight inequities, violations, and having our needs blocked. It's our most effective tool to mobilize action against injustice and harm. The biggest obstacle to social change is not heated opposition, but apathy. And yet society has conditioned many of us to suppress our anger, especially those who most deserve to feel it.

The alarms of anger and resentment are essential signals to motivate change. When we pick up subtle cues that our boundaries are being crossed, the resentment alarm shouts out loud and clear before we even have time to reflect on the situation. This alarm screams, *PROTECT YOURSELF!*

In fact, anger and resentment might be our superpower to give us the capacity to extend more compassion toward others. University of Houston researcher Brené Brown teaches that a prerequisite for compassion is healthy boundaries—defining what are okay and not okay ways for others to behave toward us. Our resentment alarms sound loudly when these boundaries need protecting. When we're unable to establish these boundaries—whether we haven't been taught to practice them or we've never been granted the power or safety to uphold them—we may armor up or burn out, reducing our capacity to maintain empathy and compassion.

For example, if someone is constantly intruding on my family time with work calls, I will resent their behavior. This resentment alarm signals to me that I need to assert the boundary of when it's okay and not okay to contact me. Then, when they approach me within these boundaries, I will have more capacity to extend attention and compassion because I'm not depleted by their behaviors. For this reason, therapist Prentis Hemphill defines boundaries as the distance you can love both yourself and others.

But our society's imbalanced structures fail to distribute power equitably, leaving too many people without the freedom and safety to act on these protective alarms. To bring our collective back to health, those of us who have been granted the power to safely express anger must use it to fight even harder for a just world for everyone, where boundaries—and all the other social privileges that impact our health—aren't just accessible to a select few.

THE COMPASS OF ENVY

Like resentment and jealousy, envy has an image problem, especially since it gained notoriety as one of Catholicism's seven deadly sins. But even envy acts as a helpful messenger.

The envy alarm signals to us that others have a reward that we need or desire. This arises from our seeking system, alerting us to what's important, with the alarm increasing in intensity when that need is unmet. When I was a medical student and resident, working sometimes up to one hundred hours a week at the hospital, I became increasingly burned-out and began to envy the patients I treated as they lay sick in their sterile beds. It sounds completely irrational to feel that way, considering those people were deeply uncomfortable, facing scary diagnoses, and wishing for nothing but a quick discharge home. But it makes sense when you see envy as a seeking signal. Envy told me that my most important and unmet need was rest, and its distress pushed me to seek it out for myself. In this way, whenever our envy alarms sound, it's helpful to ask ourselves: What need is envy highlighting for me that's both important and unmet, and how do I seek it out for myself in healthy ways?

So far, envy seems pretty harmless. The problem is that when we're overstressed or conditioned by the dynamics of dominance, our rage network may join the party in harmful ways. Rather than being inspired by the person we envy to seek out the unmet need for ourselves, we may feel an urge to destroy the thing that we envy in another.

But the mix of seeking and anger can also fuel constructive movements. Envy helps us see what needs are important and unmet, while anger motivates us to seek out justice to ensure that those needs are met more fairly. This healthy form of envy has adaptively fueled many social movements, such as Black Lives Matter and Every Child Matters, advocating for those harmed by our racist and colonial systems attain the justice and safety that white folks hold, or the Occupy movement, which fought for a more just and healthy distribution of wealth for everyone.

NO MUD, NO FLOWER

Out of the mud grows the most beautiful flower, taught Vietnamese Buddhist monk and peace activist Thich Nhat Hanh of the lotus. While our emotional signals are painful and messy, they are a magnificent alarm system to detect the imbalances in our bodies, relationships, communities, and ecosystems that, left unchecked, will make us all sick. As we're all connected within these many systems of life, we need to listen to everyone's alarms to guide our world back to health.

TWO

SELF-CARE IS COLLECTIVE-CARE

What happens to one happens to all. We can
starve together or feast together.
—ROBIN WALL KIMMERER

AS A PSYCHIATRIST, I BURNED OUT BEFORE EVERYONE ELSE. I ASSUMED I WAS TOO
weak, too soft, not made for medicine, even less suited to psychiatry.
But now I see that I was simply paying attention with an alarm system
fine-tuned to sense an imbalanced world.

In Ocean Vuong's *On Earth We're Briefly Gorgeous*, the narrator
and his grandmother watch a TV clip of a herd of buffalo running,
single file, off a cliff—"A whole streaming row of them thundering off
the mountain in technicolor."

"Why they die themselves like that?" she asked, mouth open.

"They don't mean to, Grandma. They're just following their family. That's all. They don't know it's a cliff," he responded.

"Maybe they should have a stop sign then," she said.

My burnout was a stop sign, not just for my own body to stop
in the direction it was heading, but for the larger systems I inhabit.
If you want to know how society is really doing, ask a therapist. But
we're not supposed to tell you, at least not in specific examples. Hour
after hour, we witness the harms that the imbalances in our systems
inflict on us, but we're silenced by confidentiality.

As many activists keep saying, our social structures aren't broken; they were built this way, to value profits over people, power over justice, and destruction over life. There's only so much stress we can hold until all of our systems short-circuit and collapse.

CARING FOR OUR COLLECTIVE

I once belly-flopped into the lava of American politics with an opinion piece in the *Los Angeles Times*. My inbox flooded with emails and voice messages from strangers—mostly of the all-caps-misogynistic-cursing variety. But one message diverged from this pattern, with someone writing to me, "You should lose your medical license. As a psychiatrist, you're supposed to be neutral."

To me, being apolitical when our social structures are killing us is no more neutral than standing on an empty shore and doing nothing to rescue a drowning child. As anti-apartheid activist Desmond Tutu taught, "If you are neutral in situations of injustice, you have chosen the side of the oppressor."

It's my moral duty as a physician to advocate for social change when political decisions affect our health. I refuse to spend my life bandaging wounds that could be prevented. And policies and practices that create social inequities, incite division, and devastate our environment hurt everyone's health. We *are* in this together. The injustices and destruction of our collective will poison everyone, even the most privileged bunkered away in their gated communities.

While the United States is one of the wealthiest nations in the world, with health-care spending far exceeding that of any other country, Americans experience more injuries, worse health, and shorter lives than people living in other high-income countries.[1, 2] While these health disparities most affect people from marginalized groups, even advantaged Americans—those with healthy behaviors and from white, insured, college-educated, and high-income groups—have worse health outcomes than people living in comparison countries.

British social epidemiologists Richard Wilkinson and Kate Pickett studied the health of countries for decades, hoping to discover why some countries fare so differently from others. They kept finding that the usual suspects of individual health behaviors didn't explain the health gaps. Japan, the nation with the longest life expectancies, for example, has one of the highest rates of smoking in high-income countries, with its men smoking more than twice as much as those in the US.[3] Instead, Wilkinson and Pickett found that the health of our nations is most impacted by social factors at a population level. The biggest culprit they discovered? Social inequities.[4]

When they graphed twenty high-income nations' health and social problems against their level of income inequality, they understood why the US struggles with such poor social and health outcomes, despite its total wealth and health spending. Their extensive follow-up studies and reviews proved that the level of inequality in communities and nations directly caused poor health for everyone.[5]

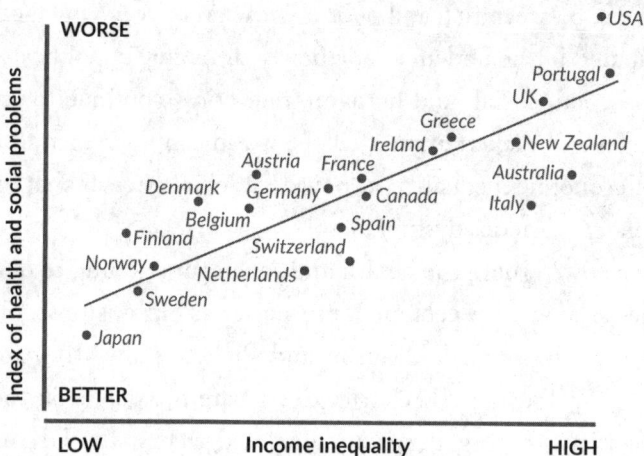

Simone Schenkman and Aylene Bousquat, researchers at the School of Public Health at the University of São Paulo, included low- and mid-income countries in their own large study of the impacts of inequality in 2021. They discovered that countries with the most inequities in not only income but also in education and health care had the worst health outcomes, regardless of the country's wealth. The authors concluded that policies that lead to inequality are "a disastrous political choice for society."[6]

Living in an inequitable country doesn't only affect those with the least privilege; it harms those with the most, too.[7] Social inequities lead not only to poor physical health outcomes and lower life expectancies for everyone, but also to higher levels of stress, mental illness (three times the rate of more equitable countries), substance use, crime, incarceration, segregation, social distrust, disrespect, violence, and lack of innovation.[8] As inequities also erode social cohesion, we isolate and engage less in politics and fixing the system's wider problems, making it harder to get ourselves out of this mess.

"The evidence that large income differences have damaging health and social consequences is already far stronger than the evidence supporting policy initiatives in many other areas of social and economic policy," say Wilkinson and Pickett. And yet politicians continue to allow the gap between rich and poor to grow every year, which can only be attributed to the undemocratic power of money in politics. As our environmental, social, and humanitarian crises continue to escalate, Wilkinson and Pickett argue that the world can no longer afford the costs of economic inequality, a "powerful social stressor that increasingly renders societies dysfunctional."[9]

Even if we ignore the health and social functioning of our communities and only see economic prosperity as our goalpost, inequality destroys that, too, Wilkinson and Pickett show. They founded the Equality Trust, a UK charity to educate the public on the costs of inequality. The organization calculated that if the UK reduced its income disparities to the lower rates of Denmark, Finland, Belgium, Norway, and the Netherlands, for example, it could save over £128 billion a year as a result of its citizens living more years in full health, better mental health, and reduced rates of homicide and incarceration.[10]

While doctors are told to "stay in your lane" and out of politics, our health depends more on public policy and practices at a population level than on our individual medical practices. We doctors take an oath to honor the health of those we serve, prevent illness whenever we can, and first do no harm. So now, more than ever, the interconnected health of our wider systems *is* our lane.

HEALTH IS BALANCED SYSTEMS

It's not only the distribution of wealth among the members of our society that needs to be in balance to sustain our health. We're all active members of many systems whose stability depends on balance.

Our world is a complex web of relations, with interdependent parts organized into multiple systems, from cells to organisms, social systems, and ecosystems. In the past three billion years of evolution, our ecosystems learned how to best organize themselves to develop sustainably and maintain balance. It's only been us humans defying these rules that's messed everything up. But it's not simply the arrival of humans to the scene that derailed its natural order. The pathology itself is a specific mindset ruled by domination, division, and indifference, when humans fail to understand their interdependence with the very systems they keep destroying.

In my home of North America, Indigenous communities lived in balance with the land for over twenty thousand years. Family physician Dr. Ojistoh Kahnawahere Horn, the president of the Indigenous Physicians Association of Canada, explains how her Kanienkehaka people's worldview centers on respecting the reciprocal relationships among all the parts of Creation. "All the beings of Creation were placed on this Earth with their own Original Instructions," she says. "We, the People, have the responsibility to steward the land, allowing for all parts of Creation to carry out those instructions, to live harmoniously, to not take more than we need, to keep the great balance, the great homeostasis, the great peace." The Haudenosaunee people, for example, guided their decisions by their Seventh Generation Principle to ensure their actions supported the health of those living seven generations in the future.

Horn speaks of her culture's traditional legal framework, which values equity and views land as shared property for communal use, not something to conquer and amass or destroy with overextraction. One example she gives is the Dish with One Spoon treaty between the Haudenosaunee and the Anishinaabeg, in which they agreed to share the lands and waters for hunting, trapping, fishing, and gathering so individual groups could not hoard or stop others from accessing them.

These Indigenous communities traditionally followed what scientists would later identify as the key principles of ecological systems theory. They gathered resources in sustainable and equitable ways that maintained the world's biodiversity by acknowledging their interdependence with all of its parts, as opposed to capitalism's goal of unlimited economic growth, which ignores our impact on the living systems around us. When hunting or farming, Indigenous communities attended to their impact on their natural environments and moved between different areas to allow the parts of the system they harvested to rebound and recover fully from their activity.[11]

Rob Kelly, an Indigenous planning and environmental manager, joined the outdoor survival contest and reality TV series *Alone Australia* only to leave the show after two days. In this show, ten contestants are dropped off miles away from anyone else, with minimal survival equipment to build their own shelter and harvest food and water, fighting to overcome both the elements and starvation to outlast the others. Kelly soon realized that winning the competition didn't align with his Indigenous values of interconnectedness. He lacked meaning without his family and felt troubled by his impact on the depleted natural world surrounding him.

Kelly explained that the traditional Indigenous people of the location, the palawa of lutruwita (Tasmania), would not stay on lands that had such exhausted resources. They would seasonally move to more hospitable locations. The mindset of the show, he continued, "immediately positions [nature] as your enemy, something to fight against, to resist. The last person standing is ultimately which person can resist what [nature] is telling them." It's counterintuitive, he argued, and the "complete opposite" to what his ancestors would have done, which would have been to listen to the feedback that the natural world provided and ensure the health and relationships of all the parts of the web of life.

This man-versus-nature mindset came on the boats of some of my own European ancestors, who forcefully displaced these sustainable Indigenous systems with their colonial culture of divide and conquer. As they failed to understand their connection to the interdependent living systems that we all depend on to survive, they began sentencing the planet to our present crisis of climate collapse and conflict. Colonists chose to violently dominate over the Indigenous stewards of the land (and, in many regions, over the Africans they enslaved to work it). They created an artificial caste system based on their own false superiority of race, subordinating and silencing those who held the knowledge and experience that they needed to survive.

The colonists replaced Indigenous governance systems with their own flawed rule of law and forced Indigenous children into residential schools to sever their connection to their communities and culture. They removed Indigenous people from stewarding their land and relocated them to small designated territories. Confined to one place, Indigenous communities could no longer practice their sustainable harvesting techniques that kept the ecosystem in balance, forcing them into poverty and illness. Nor could they continue to protect the stolen lands from the colonist's overextraction beyond the boundaries of these reserves. The colonists' actions continue to devastate not only the health and safety of Indigenous communities to this day, but that of settlers, too, as the colonists' enduring culture of domination, division, and indifference keeps destroying the entire living system that we depend on to survive, leaving the entire planet in need of life support.

"It is important to understand that colonization is not a single event in the past, but a continuous process that carries on today; one that has brought and continues to bring devastation to both our people and the environment," wrote Jennifer Grenz, a Nlaka'pamux ecologist who runs the Indigenous Ecology Lab at the University of British Columbia, in *Medicine Wheel for the Planet.* The colonial worldview, she reminds us, "gives people dominion over the other creatures of the Earth and objectifies what is referred to as 'the environment' as if it is independent from humans." She continues:

> Our Indigenous view does not allow for such separation. Our very existence is inside the ecosystem as an equal relation, meaning we are just as important as the grasshoppers, worms, birds, and soils are. Yet we find ourselves living in a world hampered by colonial legacies that continue to force us outside the ecosystem.

As the window to save our planet from environmental collapse closes, we can urgently return to the shared teachings of both the natural world's ecology and the Indigenous stewards of the land, whose tried-and-true strategies kept our ecosystems in balance long before we disrupted their course. Luckily, we already have a road map.

WE'RE ALL CONNECTED

Borders are those invented lines drawn with ash on
maps and sewn into the ground by bullets.
—Mosab Abu Toha

As humans, we can't exist isolated from the other parts of the many systems we inhabit. Many Indigenous groups across Africa describe the ethic of Ubuntu: *"I am because we are."*[12] In Xhosa, Ubuntu is translated as *"Together, we make one another human."*[13]

The first principle of both ecological systems and many Indigenous teachings around the world is how we're all mutually interdependent.[14] We shift our perspective from parts to the whole, from objects to their many relationships, from a linear model of cause and effect to the unpredictable ripples of multiple feedback loops within complex networks of life, where altering one part or linkage in the system impacts the whole in a myriad of ways.[15]

As a result, we have both differentiated and linked selves, teaches Dan Siegel, a psychiatrist and researcher at the University of California, Los Angeles (UCLA). We inhabit a body that we traditionally define as me. But our body is an open system, constantly communicating through invisible links to its environment. There is no us and them. We're all intimately connected.

Physicists now know that we live in two realms that correspond to both of these selves. First, our embodied self is a discrete entity inhabiting the material realm, in the world that we can see and touch. And we also live in the quantum realm, with invisible energy flowing through entangled webs of relationships, where parts can only be understood through their connections to the whole.

If one of the interconnected parts of a complex system acts like it doesn't belong to the system, "it will behave in a disconnected way, interdependence will shut down, and the whole complex system will lose its ability to adapt and learn," explains Siegal.[16] "In medicine, when this happens to renegade cells in the body that grow without regard to the complex living somatic system, we call it cancer."

Cancer cells are colonists who rule by supremacy, capitalists who follow the misguided principle of unlimited growth. Their marked individualism robs them of the foresight that they are trashing their own home. As they intrude on the delicate balance of their environment by exerting dominance and extracting more than their share of resources, the starved and displaced indigenous cells can no longer function to keep the system alive. Until the cancer is contained, no amount of self-care from the other body cells is going to save their lives.

While the exquisite harmony of the trillions of cells that come together to function as our bodies can be defeated by a few power-crazed cancer cells, the other living systems we inhabit are equally vulnerable to the same pathology. When the dynamics of domination corrupt our larger systems by severing our links, overextracting resources, and failing to share, we humans can become the cancer. If even a minority of us intrude on our living systems' natural balance in this way, the whole world can struggle to right itself back to health.

The fallacy of this competitive brand of individualism, with its divide-and-conquer approach to victory, is that even when we exert power over the other members of our living systems and "win," everyone still loses. Because the victors are part of the collective they've defeated, their actions are suicidal, and they're taking everyone else down with them. No amount of charity or prayers to "those in need" will fix the imbalance if we continue to support and benefit from the disparities of power and privilege that starved our neighbors of resources in the first place. Instead, we must remove the cancer from its source—the dynamics of domination—not only for the survival of humanity but for the very planet we depend on for life.

DIVERSITY AS A SURVIVAL ADVANTAGE

At one of Dan Siegel's courses, I sat drinking tea with a new friend, a fellow mindfulness-based therapist whom we all called Sparkles, as she radiates the most magnetic warmth even from a distance. Luckily, she interpreted my stalking behaviors as endearing and allowed me to starfish to her side for the week.

"Dan's brain is just so beautiful," I gushed to her, inspired by his deep understanding of all the intersections of science and psychology. "And also, I'm thrilled he's spent all this time with physicists and neuroscientists so we don't have to. It's like he's a brain cell of the system and we're heart or muscle cells, carrying his learnings to other parts of the system."

In medical school, I used to always giggle as every subspecialist addressing our lecture hall argued that their organ of expertise was the *most important* part of the body. But they're all equally important in different ways. Without any one of our unique organs, we could die, even if we had six perfect hearts to replace all the other organs. The same is true for all the members of our living systems: every diverse part is necessary to survive.

The moment I talk about moving from self-care to collective-care, many people in the West cringe, calling me a "commie," as they picture government-controlled masses in drab, shapeless clothing conforming to the same ideas, working the same jobs, and eating the same food in the same living quarters. But I see collective-care as a Pride parade, where we come together, each sparkling in our own uniquely fabulous ways, celebrating the strength of our diversity with an "anything goes" attitude—as long as our actions don't harm the collective. Botanist Robin Wall Kimmerer best illustrates this with the social structure of her Potawatomi Nation in *Braiding Sweetgrass,* where each member is responsible for cultivating their individual gifts for the purpose of giving them back for the greater good.

In fact, the rules of ecology demand this diversity for the system to survive. Ecology's second principle is that a system becomes more resilient by increasing the diversity of its individual parts, with each functioning in different yet overlapping ways.[17] We optimize our collective's health when we maximize both the diversity of the different species in our ecosystem and the specific traits of individuals within each species. By varying in biological, cultural, political, spiritual, occupational, and all the multitude of other potential differences we offer, our collective has access to more unique approaches and perspectives that can protect us from the wide spectrum of threats we face.[18]

While the value of diversity, equity, and inclusivity (DEI) is still debated by those who benefit from their positions of dominance, research in numerous fields clearly shows that diversity in a system improves it. Even in the financial realm, when McKinsey & Company evaluated data from 1,265 companies in twenty-three countries from six global regions, they confirmed in their 2023 report *Diversity Matters Even More* that companies committed to diversity perform best. Teams scoring high in ethnic diversity had a 39 percent greater likelihood of outperforming the competition, as did teams scoring high in gender diversity. On the other hand, teams scoring low in both gender and ethnic diversity were 66 percent less likely to outperform the competition.

The problems of lack of diversity is why incest is a widespread cultural taboo. When two genetically alike individuals inbreed, their offspring are susceptible to a large host of diseases caused by having too similar a genetic makeup. But when we mate with a person who's different from us, the odds of having an adaptive gene to overcome less adaptive ones are high, just as we have more varied strategies to protect our systems from a wide spectrum of threats when we vary our membership.

Yet rather than seeing diversity as a strength, we might fear it and choose to cluster with those who look, think, and act like us. We divide into opposing camps that no longer link and support the whole, cornered into yesterday's close-minded perspectives that can't adapt to today's new challenges.

"Supporting diversity is not only the right thing to do, but the smart thing to do," Michelle Bachelet, the first female president of Chile and past United Nations High Commissioner for Human Rights, shared with our group of NGO delegates at the UN Commission on the Status of Women in 2025. Loyalty is not about others agreeing with your point of view, Bachelet explained. To succeed, we need to trust others to help us see beyond our limited lenses to understand problems from many perspectives.

Social psychologists describe the problem of *groupthink*, where a group chooses the comfort of conformity and false certainty over the independent thinking and innovation required to solve new problems. Yale psychologist Irving Janis identified groupthink as the perpetrator of many foreign-policy disasters, such as the United States' failed Bay of Pigs invasion of Cuba and the Japanese attack on Pearl Harbor.[19]

We're seeing groupthink play out today in our divisive politics as online communication isolates us even further into echo chambers of confirmation bias, where we only hear ideas consistent with our in-group and villainize and dehumanize those we deem different. While social media was designed to connect us, a brief scroll through the comments section proves that it can also be weaponized to divide us, destabilizing our entire social system as our collective spirals into a combat zone.

When this division and infighting happens in our body system, we call it an autoimmune disease. The body's immune cells get confused and begin attacking the body itself, believing our own cells are threats. When it happens in our social systems, the more we split off and attack what we falsely believe to be "not us," the more we're hurting ourselves. As we retreat to our own corners and dehumanize other members of our collective, it's easy to support unjust agendas that divide—and thus destroy—us all.

ALL ARE WINNERS AND ALL ARE NEEDED

The same dynamics of division and infighting even infect our mental health treatments, pushing experts to pretend that only their own approach offers the solution to our suffering, as they split off and compete against each other for profits while protecting their progress with patents. Rather than celebrating our strength in diversity, mental health providers can fracture into warring camps of pharmacotherapy, mindfulness, cognitive behavioral, psychoanalytic, somatic, interpersonal, humanistic, emotion-focused, and other therapies, each with their own catchy acronym, like CBT, DBT, ACT, EFT, and IPT. Inside each camp, even smaller groups brand their techniques as uniquely

marketable packages, such as mindfulness-based cognitive therapy
(MBCT), mindfulness-integrated CBT (MiCBT), mindfulness-based
stress reduction (MBSR), and so on. With more than five hundred
mental health models out there, including eighty-six evidence-based
treatments listed by the American Psychological Association alone,
the mental health field may be advancing in creative solutions, but it
feels more fragmented and contentious than ever.

We can't even agree on whether being "evidence-based" is helpful.
Our inability to measure social context and the complexity of the interdependent systems we inhabit makes it hard to generalize any "evidence" to real life. Can we really measure how our treatments affect
the intricacies of our bodies, minds, and souls, especially when these
bodies, minds, and souls live in dynamic environments that constantly
affect them? As Octavia Butler explained, "All that you touch you
change; all that you change, changes you." We can't isolate the impact
of any intervention from the unexpected ripples that each small movement in our complex systems creates in faraway places.

As a clinical professor of medicine at the University of British
Columbia, I teach my students to make evidence-based clinical decisions with caution, as the evidence for many of our treatment options
follows the linear cause-and-effect models of classical research that
doesn't account for the complex systems that we all inhabit. Traditional research hopes to isolate the true effects of the single thing
we study by removing the "confounding variables" from its real-world
context. But as everything is entangled within the complex systems
we inhabit, this approach also impairs our ability to apply these findings to the real world. Complex problems like our inflamed bodies
and world require complex solutions that see the larger systems that
impact us all in a multitude of ways.

"But if everything is connected to everything else, how can we
ever hope to understand anything?" systems theorists Fritjof Capra
and Pier Luigi Luisi ask in *The Systems View of Life*. "Since all natural

phenomena are ultimately interconnected, in order to explain any one of them we would need to understand all the others, something which is not possible," they continue. "Science can never provide any complete and definitive understanding."

For this reason, health care is adopting a systems approach to studying our interventions, embracing context rather than trying to control for its effects. We realize that we can't easily predict how a complex system will behave, and that outcomes are specific to their unique context and not easily generalizable to others. We remain humble to the unintended consequences that one intervention can create in other parts of the system, a concept popularized by the Butterfly Effect, where a small change, such as a butterfly flapping its wings, in one part of a complex system can create a tornado of large changes in another. When we try to heal any of our complex systems, from our inflamed bodies to our ecosystems and the many social systems within them, we can't understand any of the parts without positioning them within the context of their interconnected whole.

Even what we define as "disordered" is decided by the cultural context of the norms and values of the time and place of which we live and is widely disputed. As part of Western psychology's dark past, David Barlow, professor emeritus at Boston University, who has written over six hundred scientific articles in the field, researched conversion therapy, what he describes as the "most regrettable initiative in my clinical research career." Queer love was falsely considered a disorder at the time. "Out of extreme pressures from society and the associated stigma, these individuals sought out treatment," says Barlow. "So very few clinicians even gave it a second thought.

"Looking back on that period from today's vantage point it is very hard to even conceive how we could not have realized the inherent conflicts in attempting to treat harmless consenting adult behavior involving love and affection," he said. Barlow learned that it's not our patterns of behaviors, thoughts, and feelings that are problematic, but how society interpret these experiences through the lens of our "continually shifting landscape of cultural values."

We've seen these norms and values decide whether the ways we express emotions, relate to one another, or think and behave are deemed "dysfunctional" or not. Is the withdrawal that arises with low mood disordered if it's an adaptation to being stuck in a toxic environment? Is the use of psychedelics "drug abuse" if it's a spiritual or healing practice? Is our escalating anxiety, rage, or grief problematic as we approach the collapse of our climate or witness civilians being murdered by the very institutions that are supposed to keep us safe? Often our experiences themselves aren't the problem; it's the society around us that rejects their diverse expressions, such as the beauty of sharing love or the value of feeling appropriate distress signals when in danger.

Diagnoses can at times feel arbitrary, then, when mental health experts divide us into one-size-fits-all disorders and offer specific treatment protocols for each silo. Mental health diagnoses are clusters of symptoms lumped together into categories listed in the *Diagnostic and Statistical Manual of Mental Disorders* (*DSM*) to help us communicate an understanding of how our distress is expressed, not precise disease processes. Splitting people into tidy little silos, each with their simple theory of cure, doesn't capture the complexity of our mental health, nor does it clarify how to heal our suffering. While diagnoses describe patterns of surface-level symptoms, we also need to look deeper to identify the underlying causes of the distress.

Unlike the flu, where a single virus creates similar symptoms in each of us, mental health conditions arise from the accumulation of a wide variety of stressors—whether biological, psychological, environmental, social, political, evolutionary, or spiritual—interacting with a wide variety of environmentally-adapted genes to dysregulate our systems into a wide variety of imbalances in our bodies, minds, and souls. As we will discuss in the next chapter, there isn't one cause, nor is there one cure.

Despite the decades of research comparing one theory of psychotherapy with another, study after study shows the same thing: they're all pretty much equally effective. This has become known as the *Dodo bird verdict*, named after the Dodo bird in *Alice's Adventures in Wonderland*, who proclaimed, "Everybody has won and all must have prizes."

During my training, University of British Columbia researcher and psychiatrist W. John Livesley taught us that since we've already established how the different approaches of psychotherapy have similar outcomes in treating mental health challenges, we can now move our efforts away from comparing each approach against each other to exploring how to combine their diverse parts.

Silos aren't bad: specialization and expertise usually deliver progress, especially in complex systems like mental health. But we need the silos to communicate with each other. Our systems are healthiest when our diverse parts link up and work together to offer unique strategies for the common good. While we may ground our approach in common principles known to be shared and effective in all therapies, we can also combine specific techniques to offer each of us a tailored assortment of strategies to meet our unique needs and contexts.[20] Just like with our other systems, we want to celebrate our diverse parts and link them together to support the health of the whole.

This echoes the reformed approaches of Stefan Hofmann and Steven Hayes, who started out as prominent figureheads in two opposing camps of therapy, cognitive behavioral therapy (CBT) and acceptance and commitment therapy (ACT). After a "stormy beginning with countless heated debates" akin to "boxing matches," they came together to take down the walls between the divided groups and create a new paradigm.[21] Their integrative process-based therapy (PBT) moves away from dividing us into specific disorders with narrow one-size-fits-all protocols to linking all of our learning to address each of our own complexities within the situational and historical contexts of our lives.

They break down their approaches into common processes that include cognitive, behavioral, somatic, social, motivational, emotional, epigenetic, neurobiological, and evolutionary factors. Then they offer whatever tool within these areas could uniquely help each of us, re-gardless of school or diagnosis.

David Barlow similarly updated his approach to create the *Unified Protocol for the Transdiagnostic Treatment of Emotional Disorders*. It's a mouthful, I know, without the sexy simplicity and branding of other approaches. But his research proves that offering a tool kit with many different resources, regardless of how one's suffering presents, is just as effective as dividing people into silos and offering diagnosis-specific tools.[22]

Even these strategies are limited by their grounding in the dominant paradigms of Western psychology, culture, and scientific methods, excluding other ways of knowing, including the abundance of rich teachings from many other cultural, spiritual, land-based, oral, and intuitive practices. Robin Wall Kimmerer uses the approach of braiding, weaving together multiple ways of knowing alongside each other—as differentiated and linked parts—without needing them to meld into one objective or universal truth. Simplicity is a fantasy, as our living systems are complex networks of many strands each holding unique truths. When we abandon the myth of certainty that pushes us to oversimplify our reality, we can embrace the many truths offered to us from teachings across cultures, disciplines, and lived experiences, all at the same time.

"The world we want is one where many worlds fit," offered the Zapatistas movement in Mexico, inspiring us to open our minds and hearts to the boundless possibilities of healthier ways of living, each adapted to our unique histories, cultures, biology, and environments.

RESTORING BALANCE TO OUR SYSTEMS

Caring for our collective doesn't take away from our freedom. It's not about conforming to the group or repressing our individual needs and desires. Our systems depend on us maintaining our freedom to stand alone at times so that groupthink doesn't weaken our capacity to offer diverse views to adapt to new challenges.

Collective care is simply recognizing that the healthiest living systems consist of diverse parts that work together to create a whole that's greater than the sum of its parts. It's knowing that we belong to something bigger than ourselves and honoring all of our important differences and relationships to this web of life so that we can be healthy because all the parts of our systems are healthy. As Audre Lorde explained, "It's not our differences that divide us. It is our inability to recognize, accept, and celebrate those differences."

While self-care is important, we need to care for both our embodied self and our collective self to ensure the health of all its connections and parts. If we stray too far into individualism, we deny our interdependence. And if we stray too far into collectivism, we may force conformity and intolerance of difference.

I wish I could offer you a one-size-fits-all approach, a simple cure to soothe all of our suffering. Of course, we dream of discovering *the* absolute truth, the secret to happiness or health or however we each define wellness. Yet we are all so beautifully diverse that we don't even share the same values and endpoints to aim our efforts. Can we both embrace the comfort that we are all in this human collective together and also cherish that we each inhabit bodies that carry specific adaptations to our unique environments and cultures, with diverse values and goals?

As the world feels more divisive than ever, recognizing our common humanity and needs is essential to compassion and connection. At the same time, Zen teacher Shunryu Suzuki worried that an emphasis on our oneness is only a one-sided understanding. "Oneness is valuable, but variety is also wonderful," he wrote in *Zen Mind, Beginner's Mind*.

There is no one path to health any more than there is one path to suffering. I hope to give you all the opportunity to collect and adapt as many strategies as you find helpful to craft personalized mental health survival kits so we can strengthen our capacity to heal together. I imagine the survival kits you create will be both as alike and different as all the experiences you've each lived. And that's wonderful.

THREE
A WORLD INFLAMED

We become inflamed when we are in abusive relationships
with our soils, our rivers, our microbial passengers, our
animal and plant relatives, our air, and each other.
—RUPA MARYA AND RAJ PATEL

———————

IN MEDICAL SCHOOL, WE LEARNED OF RISK FACTORS FOR ILLNESSES. BEING INDIGENOUS,
for example, is a risk factor for a wide variety of health problems, from
Type 2 diabetes to depression. We would tick off the box in our mental algorithm, as if being Indigenous itself were the cause of the risk.
But vulnerability to these health conditions is not an inherent characteristic of being Indigenous. Instead, we can explain most health
disparities between certain cultural, racial, gender, or class groups as
arising from the intersecting imbalances in our larger systems, such
as our uneven exposures to colonization, discrimination, violence, and
environmental toxins, and access to food, shelter, health care, employment, and education.

"To wonder why some things settle in some bodies and not others
is to begin to ask questions about power, injustice, and inequity," says
Rupa Marya, a physician at the University of California, San Francisco, and Raj Patel, a public health researcher at the University of
Texas, in *Inflamed: Deep Medicine and the Anatomy of Injustice.*

We only need to look to the COVID-19 pandemic for hard evidence
of the devastating impact of these imbalances in our systems. "Black,
Indigenous, and people of color (BIPOC) were over-represented, their

bodies subject to inflammation of all kinds, long before the SARS-CoV-3 virus ever settled into their lungs . . . Not only the lack of access to health care, but systemic social and economic disenfranchisement rendered their bodies more susceptible to Covid when it hit," Marya and Patel explain. "What this means is that the health disparities we see globally along the color lines are driven not by biological difference between fictional races but by the realities of racism." As Ta-Nehisi Coates reminds us, "Race is the child of racism, not the father."

We can't solve problems that we don't see. And when it comes to our physical and mental health, the problems that make us sick arise largely outside of the individual bodies we study and treat. Severe Covid and other chronic health conditions most impact marginalized groups because of the cumulative burdens of toxic stress, whether chemical, biological, social, psychological, ecological, political, or historical, say Marya and Patel. And the majority of these stresses are involuntary. No amount of "self-care" or individual treatment plans can overcome the weight of living in imbalanced systems.

Yet we so often blame ourselves or others for poor health. Perhaps it helps us sleep at night to think we're healthy because of our own merits, rather than unfairly hoarded privileges. Or maybe we feel more empowered if we believe that it's our own fault that we're sick, because then it's within our control to fix it, even if the added burden of stigma and blame harms us even more.

The only thing harder than recognizing and holding empathy for the unjust distribution of toxic stress that hurts the health of others is carrying these toxins in our own bodies. Inequality hurts us all, but it gravely harms the health of those who are most marginalized by our dominant society.

HOW STRESS TURNS TO DISEASE

The final principle of ecological systems is that healthy systems are flexible, regulated by intricate linkages that sense disruption and then dynamically adapt to right themselves back into balance. Our systems are resilient to short bouts of stress, with self-correcting mechanisms (known as *negative feedback loops*) that work to return the system to its natural state of equilibrium. But when these corrective mechanisms are severed or stressed to the extreme, the system loses its ability to regulate itself back to health. Instead, it shifts into self-reinforcing *positive feedback loops* that spiral the system toward escalating disorder and disease.

Our body systems are always working behind the scenes to right themselves back to balance. Our first line of defense is our interconnected immune, hormone, and nervous systems, which quietly try to reestablish balance from the inside. When this isn't enough to compensate for a disruption, our louder emotional alarms come on to push us to fix the problem from the outside. Our anger tells us to assert healthy boundaries, our fear tells us to flee from the stressor, or our hunger tells us to seek out food.

Remember how we're equipped with seven brilliant subcortical circuits that help us keep our systems in balance?

Our systems depend on us listening to the alarms of these self-corrective circuits to solve the problems that are disrupting our system's balance. And yet we often mistake the discomfort of the alarm itself as the problem, rather than the real problems that they are helping

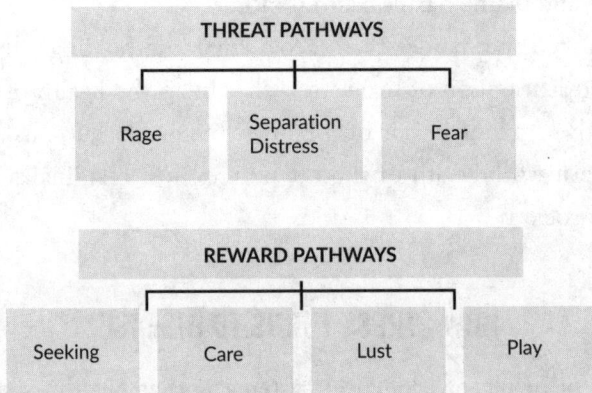

THREAT PATHWAYS

Rage	Separation Distress	Fear

REWARD PATHWAYS

Seeking	Care	Lust	Play

Seven Subcortical Threat and Reward Systems (Jaak Panksepp)

us detect. We learn to believe that the alarm's distressing feelings are dangerous and try to numb the feelings, while ignoring the threats in our environments that they are signaling us to address.

If we can't or won't listen to these alarms—or they're still not enough to solve the problem—our third line of defense comes on: the short-circuit. This forces us to pause as even louder symptoms, such as fatigue, dizziness, gastrointestinal issues, headaches or pain, the hibernation of low mood, or a bout of debilitating anxiety, push us back into the safety of our caves. It might seem dysfunctional to short-circuit, but it's preventing our system from completely dysregulating into disorder. While it doesn't usually address the source of the problem, the short-circuit pushes the pause button to give our systems time to slow down, remove ourselves from harmful environments, and reestablish balance.

Short-circuits are meant to be brief, just as we can solve so many of our electronics problems by simply turning a machine off and then restarting it again. In this way, our systems can bounce back from temporary stress, so that even if we miss the earlier signals of a stressful time and end up short-circuiting in bed for a few days, our self-correcting feedback loops can bring our body back to health on its own. But prolonged or extreme stress switches our body into the dysregulating positive feedback loops of illness.

Steve Cole, a genomics professor at UCLA, studies how persistent stress affects our gene expression. His research shows that stress increases inflammation (our first line of defense) in our body's cells. When our system perceives danger, it sets off a stress response that signals to every tissue in our body to favor inflammation and sacrifice our immune response to get ready for a wounding injury. This is our body's self-corrective mechanism to heal the disruptive injury and return the system to balance.

Our stress system works well if what we're fighting is a brief encounter with a saber-toothed tiger, says Cole, but not the complex and persistent social stresses that we find in modern society, like inequities, conflict, and isolation. Our stress response is still stuck in the Stone Age, assuming that the most helpful response to all threats is to prepare the body for a physically wounding injury.

Yet despite modern society's many advances in medicine and technology, our subjective sense of insecurity keeps increasing, Cole told me. As a result, our stress response is constantly going off, leaving our body stuck in a state of chronic inflammation. While a brief burst of inflammation helps us repair our body in the short term, chronic inflammation damages our bodies over time, accelerating the development of chronic illness, such as cardiovascular disease, diabetes, dementia, cancer, chronic fatigue or pain syndromes, and mental health conditions.

Cole and his colleagues repeated these findings many times, identifying the cellular mechanisms of how it happens: stress consistently activates a process in our bodies that increases the expression of inflammation-promoting genes and decreases the expression of antiviral and antibody-related genes in our body tissues.[1, 2] They found this pro-inflammatory expression in people exposed to a range of environmental stressors, such as low socio-economic status and social well-being, bereavement, caregiving stress, loneliness, and traumatic experiences.

Nobel Prize–winning molecular biologist Elizabeth Blackburn joined health psychologist Elissa Epel to study how chronic stress weathers our bodies by measuring the health of our telomeres—the bits at the end of our chromosomes that protect our DNA from damage. The length of our telomeres indicates our biological age—a sign of the body's wear and tear. As we age and our cells divide, our telomeres shorten. When Blackburn and Epel looked for causes of premature aging, their research kept arriving at the same conclusion: persistent stress makes our telomeres shorten faster. And once again, one of the major stressors they identified was inequality, pushing everyone's body to decline at a faster rate.

Not only does the chronic inflammation created by persistent stress accelerate aging and illness, but the resultant accelerated aging and illness then create more inflammation, dysregulating our systems into a positive feedback loop of *inflammaging*, explains a team from the Zhejiang University School of Medicine in their 2023 scientific review of inflammation and aging.[3] This process creates a "vicious cycle" of inflammation and aging, they conclude, leading to organ damage and age-related diseases.

As we explored in Chapter One, some of us evolved to have more sensitive stress responses, what we call the sympathetic nervous system (SNS) and hypothalamic-pituitary-adrenal (HPA) axis. Having a strong stress response that triggers easily is protective for short-term survival, when we don't need to worry so much about the consequences of subjective well-being and long-term health. It's what evolutionary scientist James S. Chisholm calls the "Live fast, die young" strategy. If an environment is predicted to be dangerous, making one's life expectancy short, then investing in short-term survival makes sense. Investing in the future only pays off if we are likely to be around in the future.

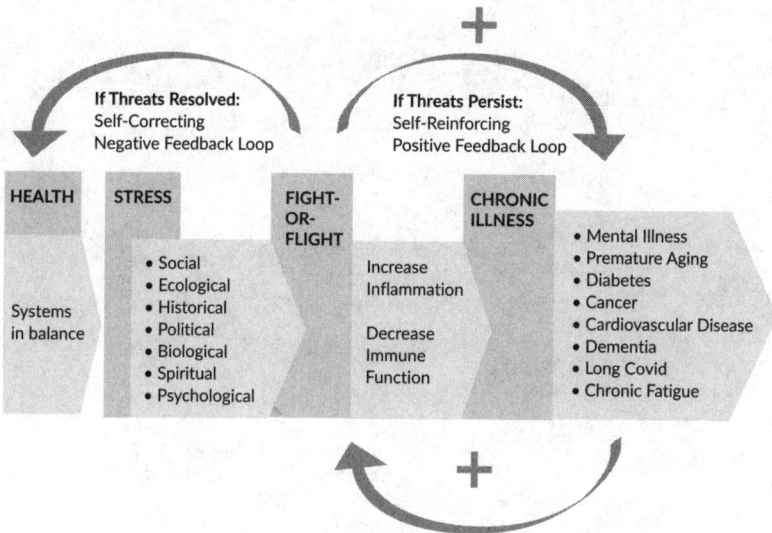

Persistent Stress Leading to the Self-Reinforcing Positive Feedback Loops of Illness

We can see the consequences of this short-term strategy in the decades of research now linking adverse childhood experiences (ACEs)—such as physical and emotional abuse, neglect, a caregiver's mental illness, and household violence—to a long list of chronic illnesses, with those experiencing the highest level of ACEs dying nearly twenty years prematurely.[4] When you add in the barrage of stresses we face every day, our bodies are often stuck in short-term survival strategies that lead to significant chronic health problems over a lifetime.[5]

Chronic exposure to stress shrinks and disrupts the communication between the neurons in our prefrontal cortex, hippocampus, and other brain regions that help us regulate our reward networks, emotions, thinking, attention, behaviors, and mood.[6] It also sensitizes our amygdala (which is responsible for our threat response) and problem-hunting default mode network, getting us stuck in unhelpful rumination about the past and future, spiraling us into more mood and anxiety symptoms, which we will discuss in later chapters.[7] Rather than righting our systems back to balance with self-correcting nega-

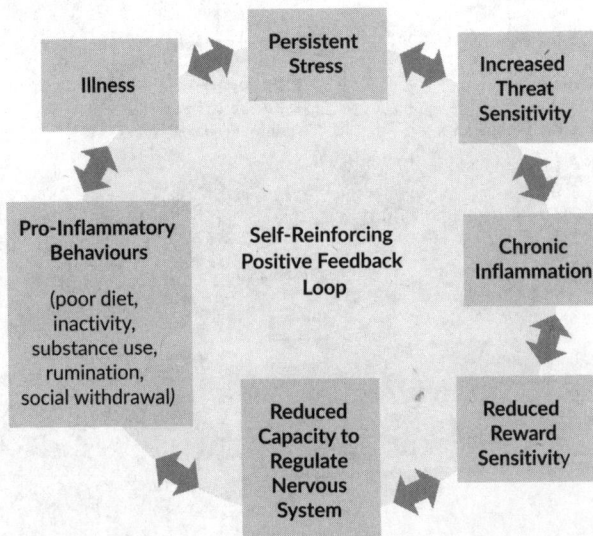

Illness

Persistent Stress

Increased Threat Sensitivity

Pro-Inflammatory Behaviours

(poor diet, inactivity, substance use, rumination, social withdrawal)

Self-Reinforcing Positive Feedback Loop

Chronic Inflammation

Reduced Capacity to Regulate Nervous System

Reduced Reward Sensitivity

tive feedback loops, persistent environmental stress pushes our body systems into the spirals of positive feedback loops, dysregulating our threat and reward networks toward escalating inflammation, unhelpful behaviors, and increasing illness.[8]

For example, if our environment becomes briefly imbalanced with too few rewards or too many threats, our emotional alarms can usually guide us away from the threats and toward more rewarding experiences. This is self-correcting because it helps us bring our systems back to balance by either decreasing the disruption of threats or meeting our needs with rewards. But unresolved stress moves our systems into positive feedback loops, dysregulating our threat and reward pathways, increasing inflammation, and promoting behaviors that keep pushing us further toward imbalance. If our alarms persistently sound with ongoing stress, our threat sensitivity increases, while our reward sensitivity decreases, pushing us into habits of retreating from our environments for prolonged periods of time, because we perceive the world to be more threatening and less rewarding.

We see this in depression, when the fish have come back after a slow season, but we are still stuck in our caves, unable to leave the safety of what was intended to be only a temporary respite. Anhedonia, a common symptom of depression, describes this state of low reward sensitivity, in which the things that used to feel rewarding no longer do, leaving us much less motivated to pursue them. When we move into the positive feedback cycle of anxiety disorders, our heightened threat sensitivity leaves us stuck in habits of avoiding and worrying about situations more than the true threat requires, so we also miss out on all the rewards in our environments.

One of my mentors, University of British Columbia researcher and professor Jehannine (J9) Austin, created the jar analogy to illustrate the complex interplay of what makes us sick and well again.[9] We're all born with a random assortment of genetic factors inherited from our parents, each with small effects that accumulate to impact our mental health. These genetic factors can be illustrated as the balls

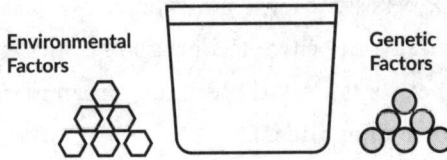

Environmental Factors / Genetic Factors

we all begin with in our jar at conception. And remember, even something as biological as our genetics is impacted by our ancestors' environments through natural selection and epigenetics.

Then, our jars fill up from the many exposures to stress in our environment over time, with each stress interacting with the others in the jar in complex ways. The jar represents the amount of stress that our system can hold and still stay regulated with its self-corrective negative feedback loops. When the jar overflows with stressors, the overwhelmed system switches to positive feedback loops of escalating dysregulation. Without our negative feedback loops to regulate us back to balance, we experience mental health symptoms that become disabling and distressing enough to be diagnosed as a mental health disorder.

To return our systems back to balance, we can work to remove some of the stress from our overflowing jars, when possible, or we can increase the height of the jar with a wide variety of strategies, such as mental health therapy and skills, medications, physical activity and diet, meditation and spiritual practices, and meaningful engagement

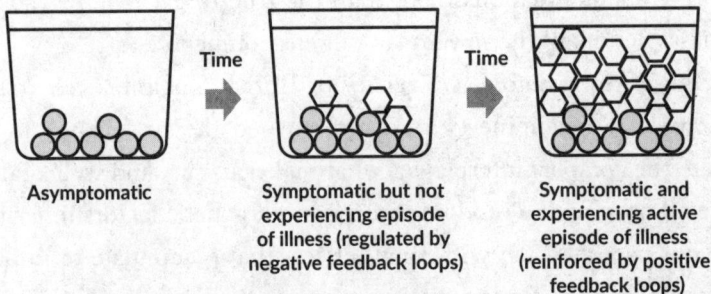

Asymptomatic

Symptomatic but not experiencing episode of illness (regulated by negative feedback loops)

Symptomatic and experiencing active episode of illness (reinforced by positive feedback loops)

and belonging to our wider systems. We can mix and match from the long list of possible strategies to bring our systems back to balance, in the same way each of us amassed a mix of many stresses to disrupt it. But we also need to address the problem from its root: the imbalances in our world that keep filling up our jars in the first place, dysregulating us all.

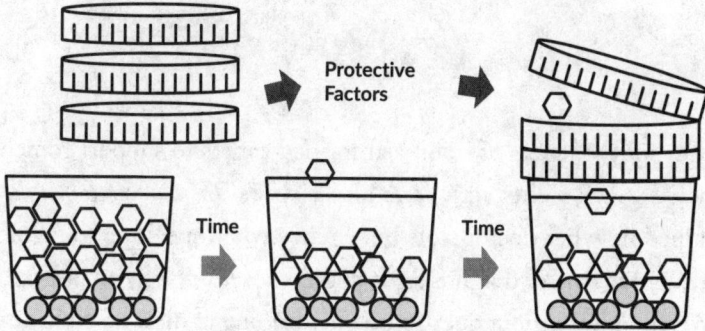

THE ABCs OF REGULATION

To bring our bodies back to balance, we can learn to pay attention to our body's helpful alarms that warn us that our jar is filling, using these messages to identify and solve the problems that they detect. The more we pay attention to our self-correcting distress signals early on and solve the problems that they signal, the less likely we'll get stuck in the escalating positive feedback loops of illness later.

When we find our system dysregulating into our stress physiology, we can rebalance our nervous systems by practicing the ABCs of regulation. In medicine, we learn about the ABCs of cardiac resuscitation, focusing on establishing an airway, breathing, and circulation. ABC can also describe what our three subcortical alarm systems of rage, separation distress, and fear need to stabilize: agency, bonding, and containment.[10] When faced with moments of feeling overwhelmed, we can resuscitate our nervous systems by regaining a sense of agency (autonomy and justice), bonding (connection and belonging), and containment (predictability and safety).

Threat Network	ABC's for Regulation
RAGE	AGENCY Sense of autonomy, boundaries, and justice
SEPARATION DISTRESS	BONDING Sense of belonging & connection, care, play, intimacy
FEAR	CONTAINMENT Sense of safety, grounding, & predictability structure, routine, & expectations

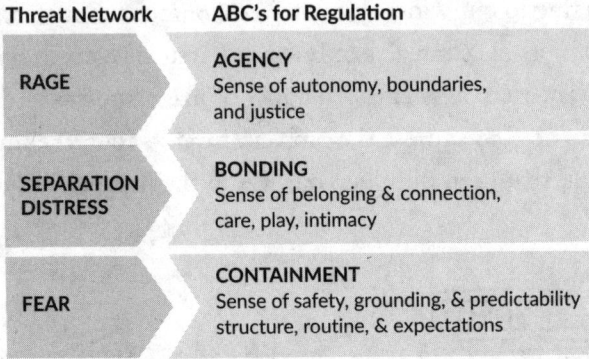

One of the tenets of trauma-informed care is to support someone's agency. In civil rights activist Audre Lorde's *The Cancer Journals*, she explained how her doctor stole her agency when speaking to her about a threatening cancer diagnosis. "If you do not do exactly what I tell you to do right now without questions you are going to die a horrible death," he told her, pushing her even further into her stress response. "What that doctor could have said to me that I would have heard was, 'You have a serious condition going on in your body and whatever you do about it you must not ignore it or delay deciding how you are going to deal with it because it will not go away no matter what you think it is,' acknowledging my responsibility for my own body," Lorde explained.

In occupational stress injuries, when traumatic events in the field push service members into a stress or trauma response, a key principle to their care is to keep them closely attached to their peers so that they continue to feel bonded as a vital contributor to the team and its mission.[11] The iCOVER protocol has been used in many areas, from combat to health care, to help members identify stress and trauma reactions in their peers, offer the distressed team member a commitment to keep them close, and then ask simple questions to ground them in the present moment, stimulate thinking, and request direct or simple actions that can restore a sense of agency and containment.[12]

The Four Rs of supporting someone with dementia who becomes

distressed and disoriented follow the same principles of the ABCs: reassure them with connection, reestablish a routine (to offer predictability and containment), reminisce to ground them in their identity and belonging, and redirect to a simple activity that brings them a sense of agency.[13]

When we feel overwhelmed by the enormity of our interconnected world crises, in some situations, we can work to decrease the danger by reducing our exposure to unsafe environments by, for example, coming together to help change our harmful systems or practicing boundaries to take respite from the toxic stress. Even when that's not possible, we can still increase our sense of inner safety by anchoring in the ABCs, that is, the bonding and belonging of others, the containment of predictable routines and rituals, and the agency of small actions that we can control, such as showing up to vote, organizing mutual aid, reducing our own carbon footprint, or supporting one specific cause or person.

In the same way, we can notice and respond to the signs of dysregulation in our larger systems: our growing inequality, divisiveness, and conflict, the fires, floods, and pandemics. These are the glaring warnings that our entire system is spiraling toward disorder. Luckily, coming together to rebalance our systems not only solves the source of our sickness, but heals our inflamed bodies while we do it.

In July 2013, when Alicia Garza, special projects director at the National Domestic Workers Alliance, learned that the courts had acquitted George Zimmerman for the murder of seventeen-year-old Trayvon Martin, she shared her anger and grief on Facebook with the hashtag #BlackLivesMatter.

Garza joined activists and community organizers Opal Tometi, the executive director of the Black Alliance for Just Immigration, and Patrisse Cullors, executive director of the Coalition to End Sheriff Violence in L.A. Jails, to launch Black Lives Matter. Cullors quickly posted a mission statement for their movement online, describing their work as "provid[ing] hope and inspiration for collective action to build collective power to achieve collective transformation, rooted in grief and rage but pointed toward vision and dreams."

Garza, Tometi, and Cullors attended to their alarms of grief, rage, and fear, and used them to motivate the adaptive response of bringing others together to fight for a healthier future for us all. This focus on contributing and caring for others is the exact antidote to the chronic inflammation of illness.

In 2015, Steve Cole began studying whether someone's sense of purpose and meaning in life could protect them against the escalating inflammation of unremitting social stress, like isolation. He had found that the stress of disconnection from others increased a person's expression of pro-inflammatory genes and decreased their expression of antiviral genes. But the effects were completely reversed when people reported having meaning and purpose in life.

Other researchers around the world confirmed that we can dampen our inflammatory stress physiology with prosocial behavior,[14] engagement with others in meaningful activity,[15] and eudaimonic well-being, which is a sense of purpose, meaning, and social embeddedness.[16]

"What seems to work best is getting people to focus on something they care about in life. Something aspirational and generative, and then getting them to collaborate with others in bringing about this desired value," says Cole. A sense of purpose shifts our brains away from our threat networks and toward our seeking and care systems—"Circuits in the brain that seem to be able to elbow aside threat signaling," he says. "So, there's something about going after what you really care about that's even more powerful than avoiding what you're afraid of."

We can switch away from our threat networks and into our reward pathways by engaging in the ABCs of regulation, and especially by focusing on collaborating in meaningful ways with others for maximum anti-inflammatory benefits.

While studies have found that these altruistic types of behaviors decrease our inflammatory stress response, focusing on self-satisfying, hedonistic types of seeking actually increases our inflammation.[17]

ABC's for Regulation

AGENCY Sense of autonomy, boundaries and justice	**SEEK**
BONDING Sense of belonging & connection	**CARE, PLAY, LUST**
CONTAINMENT Sense of safety, grounding, & predictability structure, routine, & expectations	**SEEK**

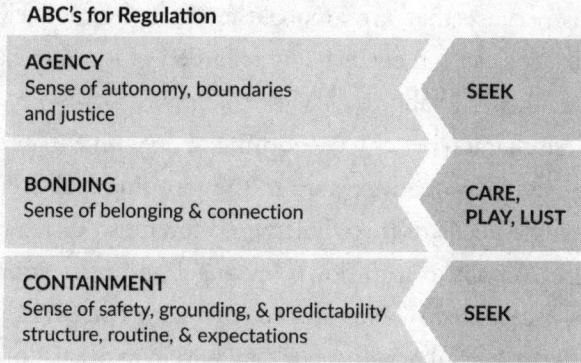

While we might feel good when consuming luxuries, this route to experiencing a sense of well-being appears to have harmful biological impacts when it predominates over altruistic behaviors. Once again, helping others helps ourselves, while hoarding privileges and satisfying only ourselves makes us sick.[18]

SMILING TO DEATH

Despite these findings, caring for our collective can't be selfless. We can stray too far toward altruism by only focusing on the needs of others while ignoring the important messages that our own body's alarms are signaling. It's all about balance. We're also a vital part of the collective we're nurturing.

Decades of research point to the same conclusion: pleasing, pushing down our emotional alarms and exclusively prioritizing only the needs of others lead to chronic illness, explains Canadian physician Gabor Maté in *The Myth of Normal: Trauma, Illness and Healing in a Toxic Culture*. Ignoring or suppressing how we feel and what we need—whether it's done consciously or unconsciously—revs up our stress response, pushing our body toward chronic inflammation and illness.

"Why these features and their striking prevalence in the personalities of chronically ill people are so often overlooked—or missed entirely," is because they are among the "most normalized ways of being in this culture, largely by being regarded as admirable strengths rather than potential liabilities," Maté told me.

Yet these characteristics have nothing to do with will or conscious choice, he says. "No one wakes up in the morning and decides, 'Today, I'll put the needs of the whole world foremost, disregarding my own,' or 'I can't wait to stuff down my anger and frustration and put on a happy face instead.'" Nor are we born with these traits. Instead, they are adaptations to preserve our connection to others, often at the expense of our health.

We develop these traits to be accepted, in what Maté describes as the tug of war between our competing needs for attachment and authenticity. We need attachment to survive, as we are a social species, wired for connection, conforming to the needs and rules of others to secure our membership in groups. But we also need authenticity to keep us healthy. Our need to belong and be accepted by others can push us to suppress these vital emotional alarms, increasing our body's inflammation while disarming our ability to protect ourselves and solve the problems of our collectives. It's no surprise, then, that those more disempowered in our societies are forced to shape and suppress their emotions and needs most gravely to survive, says Maté. This highlights the need for systemic change to fight for equity, inclusivity, and safety to improve everyone's health.

We can practice unlearning these patterns by bringing more awareness to our own emotional signals and needs, rather than automatically ignoring them in the service of others, which we will focus on in later chapters. Then we can learn to become more flexible in our responses to meet the unique needs of each situation, rather than react on autopilot with the old patterns that we learned to cope in past environments. "We might now find ourselves able to pause in the moment and say, 'Hmm, I can tell I'm about to stuff down this feeling,'" Maté says. "'Is that what I want to do? Is there another option?'"

RESISTING GRIND CULTURE

We can also miss the early warning signs of our alarms when the nonstop stress of our world punts us into a permanent state of short-circuit.

"Exhaustion keeps us numb, keeps us zombie-like, and keeps us on their clock," wrote Tricia Hersey, an American poet, theologian, and activist, in her book, *Rest Is Resistance: A Manifesto.* "I believe the powers that be don't want us rested because they know that if we rest enough, we are going to figure out what is really happening and overturn the entire system."

I discovered Hersey's work after countless friends nudged me toward her, not because they thought I'd love what she had to say, but because I urgently needed to hear it. I flipped through the pages of Hersey's book with deep discomfort. Her words were a cold shower, waking me up to the truth that the emperor I was unknowingly worshipping was not only naked but also super shady.

I had been brainwashed by the cult of productivity, equating my worth with how much I produced without question. Sure, I worked as a therapist and taught mental health workshops for a living, but I managed to even turn sharing wellness into something deeply depleting because I didn't feel I had permission to slow down.

And I was just so tired.

I *am* still so tired. I just said no to a meaningful position this morning, after two weeks of being stuck on a painfully slow Ferris wheel of indecision. The role aligned perfectly with so many of my values. And yet, my friends and therapist kept pointing out my pattern of adding on new responsibilities to my life without ever letting go of old ones, leading to perpetual overwhelm and exhaustion.

Every "yes" I say to work, my community, my friends—even when it's a "hell yes!"—is also a no to something else, maybe my loved ones or wellness, whether or not I say no out loud. And when I can't set healthy boundaries, my body will always say it for me instead. It comes out in sickness, burnout, free-floating anxiety, or shutdown.

In my case, I can't rest because a few layers below my facade of confidence, there's a lingering sense that I'm still never enough. Underneath the frantic productivity is a belief that I will be kicked out of the community if I don't contribute perfectly, that my only worth is in my service to others. And yet, the feedback I receive from my loved ones is that my excessive busyness is a barrier to belonging. My strategy to create connection impedes it.

Grind culture normalizes pushing our bodies to the brink of destruction, Hersey argues. It normalizes pushing our social systems and environment to the brink, too. It's "made us all human machines, willing and ready to donate our lives to a capitalist system that thrives by placing profits over people," says Hersey. "Rest is radical because it disrupts the lie that we are not doing enough."

Capitalism's shiny PR campaign of the fancy cars and white picket fences of the American Dream worked hard to hide its roots in the violence and theft of colonialism and slavery. In his 2019 *New York Times Magazine* article, "In Order to Understand the Brutality of American Capitalism, You Have to Start on the Plantation," Matthew Desmond, a sociology professor at Princeton University, explains, "This is a capitalist society. It's a fatalistic mantra that seems to get repeated to anyone who questions why America can't be more fair or equal."

By the eve of the Civil War, the millionaires of the Mississippi Valley, their wealth amassed off the backs of the people they enslaved to grow and pick cotton, had profited more than all the railroads and factories in the country, says Desmond. The cotton plantation was America's first big business, with bosses sacrificing their humanity for profits, squeezing maximum productivity out of the people they enslaved. Desmond continues:

If today America promotes a particular kind of low-road capitalism—a union-busting capitalism of poverty wages, gig jobs and normalized insecurity; a winner-take-all capitalism of stunning disparities not only permitting but awarding financial rule-bending; a racist capitalism that ignores the fact that slavery didn't just deny black freedom but built white fortunes, originating the black-white wealth gap that annually grows wider—one reason is that American capitalism was founded on the lowest road there is.

That's why Tricia Hersey refuses to participate in this system. The biggest obstacle to rest, though, she teaches, is that we have been socialized to believe in a model of scarcity. She understands the need to pay the bills, and at the same time, she challenges us to imagine rest in a new way: as a mind shift, a slow and consistent practice, filled with grace, using every tool we have to constantly repair what grind culture has done to us. We can shift our values away from the overconsumption and extraction of finite resources and toward the infinite abundance of love and time and wellness. "To declare to the systems, 'No, you can't have me. My body belongs to me. I will never donate my body to grind culture. I will rest,' is a bold political statement against a system that has used bodies as a tool for oppression for centuries," she continues.

Culture change comes from people collectively seeing the problem and then revolting against it, especially those of us whose power and privilege creates and reinforces it. We can all explore our different roles and responsibilities for rebelling against this toxic mode of existence as we U-turn to a healthier path.

Last night, as I continued to tangle myself into a net of doubt around how to proceed with this new opportunity, my dear friend asked me, "What if you were already enough without this position? What decision would you make?"

"I would choose to rest," I said.

So, I declined the role.

And yet my inherited privileges give me the freedom to make choices that so many don't possess. How can we share the Earth's resources and dismantle these harmful systems that drive our grind culture so that everyone can choose to step off the toxic treadmill, not just a lucky few?

We can't be well if the very foundation we've built on is rotten. We're simply repainting the walls a pretty color, knowing that the house could collapse at any moment because its weight is wobbling on unbalanced structures. True wellness requires a rebalancing of our entire system, rebuilding it on a sustainable, equally distributed foundation.

AN INFLAMED PLANET

There's a growing trend I see in my clinic every day that wasn't covered in my training. Once we work through the acute fires of what brings people to my office, a deeper sadness, a helplessness—really, an existential crisis—unravels: ecological grief and anxiety. *What's even the point of it all if our entire species will soon be extinct?*

I feel it, too, daily. I'm right there with them, facing the increasingly spoken alarms of grief, rage, guilt, and fear that we have destroyed our world so brutally that our children and grandchildren's lives may forever be harmed and shortened.

I first heard the term *eco-anxiety* years ago from my friend and colleague Courtney Howard, an emergency doctor working in Yellowknife, in Canada's Northwest Territories. Her own eco-anxiety pushed her to sound the alarms for planetary health back when we were in medical school together. Howard's drive only magnified after she moved to the subarctic, where her Indigenous patients talked about how their rapidly changing landscape affected their food security and physical safety. Then, upon returning home from working with Doctors

Without Borders (Médecins Sans Frontières) on a children's malnutrition project in Djibouti, Howard realized that the most impactful way to promote a healthy future for patients at home and abroad would be to work at the intersection of climate change and health.

As the international policy director for the *Lancet* Countdown on health and climate change, Howard's prescription pad is not ordering medications to treat ecological grief and anxiety. This distress is an accurate signal for danger. It's telling us that we need to act differently if we're all going to survive. Instead, she prescribes low-carbon transportation, plant-rich diets, integrating health impact evaluations into environmental assessments, fossil fuel divestment, and carbon pricing to recover the health of our planet.

Eco-activist Naomi Klein agrees. "What gets me most are not the scary scientific studies about melting glaciers, the ones I used to avoid. It's the books I read to my two-year-old son," she wrote in *This Changes Everything*. Upon the seventy-fifth reading of her son's favorite book, *Looking for a Moose,* it hit Klein—whose research had taken her to northern Alberta's tar sands, where the Beaver Lake Cree Nation told her that the moose's flesh had turned green, or more commonly, that the moose were simply gone—that her son might never get to see a moose in his lifetime.

"When fear like that used to creep through my armor of climate change denial, I would do my utmost to stuff it away, change the channel, click past it," Klein continues. "Now I try to feel it. It seems to me that I owe it to my son, just as we all owe it to ourselves and one another."

Like us, our ecosystems are resilient, having adapted to humanity's reckless assaults on its health for centuries. But their resilience is not an invitation for continued abuse. "Just because biology is full of generosity does not mean its forgiveness is limitless," Klein explains. "With proper care, we stretch and bend amazingly well. But we break too—our individual bodies, as well as the communities and ecosystems that support us."

I facilitate groups and workshops that teach mental health skills, such as mindfulness, to support our wellness so we can manage the emotional stress and pain of living in these uncertain times. Yet I'm careful to stay away from the new wave of "McMindfulness"—the idea that rather than addressing the valid problems that our emotions are signaling, we offer isolated wellness classes to build "resilience" so participants stay burning in the flames even longer without extinguishing the fires.

Instead, we must stop averting our gaze to the reality of climate collapse and use this distress to motivate action. Fear is a survival response that pushes us to flee from danger and run toward safety. "But we need somewhere to run to," says Klein. "Without that, the fear is only paralyzing. So, the real trick, the only hope, really, is to allow the terror of an unlivable future to be balanced and soothed by the prospect of building something much better than many of us have previously dared hope."

Yes, we are all facing the end of the world if we don't change our course. But Robyn Maynard, assistant professor of Black feminism at the University of Toronto and author of *Policing Black Lives*, argues that all world-endings are not tragic.[19] "In order to make earthly planetary survival possible, some versions of this world *need* to end (and indeed, should never have begun in the first instance)," she says, referring to our present epoch dominated by colonialism and capitalism that demands ongoing inequities and racial and ecological violence to survive. Can we celebrate the end of *this* world and choose a different path for a new one?

Marjorie Kelly cofounded Corporation 20/20 at the Tellus Institute, asking leaders in business, law, government, labor, and civil society to explore this question: "How could we redesign businesses to incorporate social and ecological aims as deeply as financial ones?" One day, as she taught with ecologist Stephan Harding, he completely changed her approach.[20] "You don't start with the corporation and ask how to redesign it," Harding told her. "You start with life, with human life and the life of the planet, and ask, how do we generate the conditions for life's flourishing." He continued, "A thing that is right will enhance the stability and beauty of the total ecosystem," referencing Aldo Leopold's *Land Ethic*. "It is wrong when it damages it."

Kelly took Harding's advice, and moved to The Democracy Collaborative, where she now works as a senior fellow to build a thriving democratic economy through systems change from the bottom up.[21] Their Next System Project recognizes that systemic problems require systemic solutions. To improve our economies, we must also address the deep crises of climate change, inequality, racial injustice, and our failing democracies. They're all connected.

When we try to heal our complex systems, from our inflamed bodies to our ecosystems and the many social systems within them, we can't understand any of the parts without positioning them within the context of their interconnected whole. For example, when economists try to measure development in linear ways, such as using the single economic dimension of gross domestic product (GDP), they fail to understand the economy within its larger system, such as its interrelated health, social, ecological, cultural, and spiritual functioning.[22] We can instead borrow from the field of ecology to practice sustainable development, recognizing that each dimension that we study is inseparable from the greater web of life.[23]

This is why Naomi Klein, her husband, Avi Lewis, and activists Katie McKenna and Bianca Mugyenyi organized the Leap Manifesto: A Call for a Canada Based on Caring for the Earth and One Another, a collective that began in 2015 at a meeting in Toronto attended by representatives for Canada's Indigenous rights; social and food justice; environmental, faith-based, and labor movements; and others. The Leap Manifesto started from the belief that the crises of inequality and climate change overlap, and stem from the same ailing systems. Only intersectional solutions and alliances to rebuild our broken relationships to this planet and each other will save us.

"I am convinced that climate change represents a historic opportunity," says Klein. The Leap Manifesto reasons that to tackle climate

change, we need to break it out of the single-issue silo. Climate change
demands the rebuilding of our inflamed world, from reclaiming our
democracies from corrosive corporate influences, to investing in starving public infrastructure like mass transit and affordable housing,
taking back ownership of essential services and remaking our sick agricultural systems into something much healthier, opening borders to
migrants whose displacement is linked to climate change, and true reconciliation with Indigenous peoples. We can't only resist toxic systems
and ideologies; we must also create healthier models to move toward.

We can extend the ABCs of regulation to remind us of what all
the parts of our interdependent systems need to return to balance.

ABC's for Regulation

AGENCY
Promote equity, justice, freedom, and reciprocity

BONDING
Promote diversity, inclusion, belonging, connection, reciprocity
and care for all parts of our system

CONTAINMENT
Promote safety, sustainability, structure, expectations, and balance

As a therapist, I refuse to promote tools that simply soothe our
distress so that we can "become more resilient" and continue to ignore these dire threats even longer, while silently dysregulating all of
our systems. Instead, we can equip ourselves with a variety of mental
health skills to rebuild our capacity to stay alert to these alarms and
use them to break us out of this mess. But first, we must understand
how much our past impacts our alarms today, complicating their messages by confusing past threats for those in the present.

FOUR

WE ARE OUR HISTORY

> History is not in the past. It is in the present. We
> carry our history with us. We are our history.
> —James Baldwin

I CIRCLED AROUND MOORE HALL AT THE UNIVERSITY OF CALIFORNIA, LOS ANGELES (UCLA) for the third time. Security officers blocked each entrance as police in riot gear patrolled the streets. Metal fences walled off the building from protesters, and barricades separated protesters on the left from those on the right. Everyone was preparing for Donald Trump Jr.'s arrival to promote his new book, *Triggered*.

As I approached the group of people whose politics opposed my own, my nervous system flung into fight mode. I tensed up, glaring at them, as if a different person had just grabbed the reins of my brain.

I was at UCLA to train in mentalization-based therapy (MBT) and was learning about just these kinds of moments, when stress switches off our mind's higher functions in favor of fast survival reactions. The visiting professor and codeveloper of MBT, British psychiatrist Anthony Bateman, playfully called it "boom time." In other words, we're triggered.

To mental health professionals, *triggered* describes intense emotional and physical reactions linked to past traumatic experiences, arising involuntarily from subcortical parts of our nervous systems. Our bodies suddenly jump into their fight, flight, or freeze reactions when we encounter situations that resemble ones that harmed us in the past.

Many of us now often use the concept more broadly—whether linked to personal traumatic experiences or not—to describe the activation of intense emotional reactions in response to anticipated threats. As we explored in Chapter One, our alarm systems are adaptations not only to our own exposures to traumatic experiences, but also to those inherited from our ancestors and collectives. I've yet to meet anyone whose lineage didn't face the traumas of war, violence, oppression, exploitation, or persecution. It's no surprise, then, that all our bodies and brains carry sensitive alarm systems to signal danger.

We often talk about our fight, flight, or freeze response in the face of a potential threat, but stressful experiences can first push us to fawn, when we attempt to socially engage by connecting with others to provide support, problem-solve together, or appease a potential perpetrator. If these strategies don't work, our bodies may then jump into fight or flight mode, ramping up our emotional activation to energize us to meet the challenge. We can think of these reactions in relation to our subcortical threat networks: fight relates to our rage system, flight to our fear system, and fawn to our separation distress (although fawning can also be a skillful strategy to solve the threats of our rage and fear networks). Our final resort is to short-circuit into freeze—to play dead, shut down, or numb out—a particularly helpful response when we are powerless to change the situation.

When we or our ancestors have experienced recurrent or serious threats, our nervous systems adapted by fine-tuning our alarms to be more sensitive to detecting potential threats, as we explored in the last chapters. We habitually jump into the fawn, fight, flight, or freeze reactions at the first hint of threat. Remember our brain's motto: it's better to be safe than sorry. When given the choice between activating a distressing stress response or underestimating a potential threat, those who prepare for the worst are most likely to survive.

If we've been exposed to situations of ongoing powerlessness in our pasts, we often adapt to our environments by skipping over the earlier steps in our stress response, having learned that our fawn, fight, or flight reactions are futile. For example, if our fawning responses are regularly met with hostility or apathy, we might learn to jump straight into the fight or flee response, since we learned from our earlier life experiences that cooperative tactics don't work. When we're exposed over and over to stressful situations that we have no control over, such as systemic injustices or prolonged conflict and abuse, we can adapt by jumping directly to freeze with each new stressor, checking out, feeling apathy, or shutting down. We skip over the more activating defenses of fawn, fight, or flight because we've learned from past experiences that we have no power to change the situation, no matter how hard we try.

So, when I encounter people promoting politics that strongly oppose my values, I'm flooded with a slideshow of our world's injustices that I associate with their politics, forcing me into my rage network's fight mode. I'm no longer capable of being compassionate or curious toward all the experiences that made these people who they are: humans, just like me, desperately trying to belong and survive, socialized by complex forces outside of their awareness and control, and who carry the historical trauma from centuries of conflict. (As with inflammation and illness, trauma isn't distributed equally among us. Those oppressed by others are harmed much more. Yet we'll explore in this chapter how even those in positions of dominance are harmed by the trauma dynamics of domination and subordination.)

In fight mode, rather than reflecting, acknowledging uncertainty, and responding with empathy to the complexity of the situation, we flip into the false refuge of certainty. *I know these guys—they're uncaring, misogynistic, racist fascists.* We know we're right, stick to our story, and take immediate actions to prove it. When we observe undesirable behavior in others, we too often reflexively tell them off, shaming them with the message *I'm right and you're an idiot*, the title of a 2016 book by James Hoggan on the state of today's public discourse. Then, we push them into boom time.

We temporarily fry our abilities to respond thoughtfully in favor of knee-jerk survival reactions. While we're all capable of astonishing compassion, empathy, creativity, and cooperation, the part of our brains needed for these functions—the prefrontal cortex—gets hijacked by our stress response. We cannot connect skillfully in boom time—the wall goes up and it's impossible to let anything in.

We've gotten ourselves into a self-fulfilling prophecy on a grand scale: When most everyone is dysregulated, our reactivity creates an unsafe world. And without safety, everyone gets even more dysregulated. Once again, we've shifted our systems into the positive feedback loops of escalating disorder, but this time on a societal level.

As we become more divided, the more we attack each other, the more we're left unable to truly see each other as complex human beings who have been hurt and crave safety and dignity, just like us. And the more we all lose our humanity.

Whether we like it or not, we're all on the same team, confronted by shared problems—like the collapse of our climate, global conflicts, and pandemics—that require coming together with diverse perspectives. We need to feel safe and secure enough to regulate our own nervous systems and regain balance in our collectives.

But the source of the problem isn't fragile individuals being triggered without cause, as Trump Jr. argued in his book. It's our vicious culture of domination, division, and indifference, inherited from generations of trauma on all sides, creating a domino effect of dysregulation in us all.

If we're to stop the spiral of escalating conflict in our world, we must first see the culture of trauma that we've all inherited from centuries of violence and power imbalances living in our bodies and minds today. Only through acknowledging these patterns of personal, collective, and historical trauma can we choose the freedom of a healthier path. But first, we need to see that trauma lives in everyone, and it's really dark and scary in there.

HISTORICAL TRAUMA LIVES IN US ALL

Derek Thompson - *Thlaapkiituup*, the director of Indigenous Engagement at the University of British Columbia, gave the opening speech at our annual Pacific Psychopharmacology Conference in Vancouver, BC, the day before our National Day for Truth and Reconciliation in 2023. He warned us not to diagnose mental health symptoms in Indigenous people with the dizzying array of labels from the *Diagnostic and Statistical Manual of Mental Disorders* (*DSM*), but as the "affliction of the residential school syndrome." This echoes the concept of "concentration camp syndrome," which describes the enduring challenges carried in the bodies of Holocaust survivors and their descendants.

When we think of the impacts of historical trauma, we reference the descendants of survivors of genocides, slavery, or colonialization. But we fail to acknowledge the unresolved trauma living in the bodies of the people who perpetrated and benefit from the harm.

"If First Nations people are sick," Thompson - *Thlaapkiituup* asked, "if we suffer the past in perpetual syndromes of sickness, if we pass along intergenerational trauma of the Indian residential school syndrome to our children and grandchildren, this begs the question, how sick are the people that created the Indian residential school system, and what are they doing about their sickness?"

Alok (ALOK) Vaid-Menon, author of *Beyond the Gender Binary,* reflects the same sentiment when speaking about their marginalization from not fitting into society's gender binary. "There's no such thing as transgender issues; there are issues that nontrans people have on themselves that they are taking out on us," they posted on Instagram.

In my child psychiatry rotation, we learned that the "identified patient"—that is, the one who presents to therapy with symptoms—is often the scapegoat expressing the sickness of the people in their much larger social system. As we delve into why a child is acting out or anxious, while their inherited biology sensitizes their stress responses, we may also find that a source of their symptoms is the trauma living in the bodies of their parents, who, carrying generations of historical trauma, never had the privilege of learning to care for them in a healthier way. Or perhaps it's the abuse the child faces at school arising from the trauma living in their bully's body. Or it's the adversities they constantly

face from the systemic oppression from their societies living in the bodies of those who hold power, whose political decisions reflect their own
incapacity to access trust, empathy, and compassion. If we focus only
on the identified patient, we aren't getting to the source of the problem.
We need to look upstream to treat the people and systems perpetuating
the pain if we are going to prevent it from happening again.

The root of the trauma living in the bodies of marginalized people
is the trauma living in the bodies of their oppressors, which made
them capable of committing or complicitly witnessing such crimes to
humanity, explains racial trauma expert Resmaa Menakem:

> The conflict has been festering for centuries . . . Even in the 1860s,
> these conflicts were already centuries old. They began in Europe
> during the Middle Ages, where they tore apart close to two million
> white bodies. The resulting tension came to America embedded in
> the bodies of Europeans, and it has remained in the bodies of many
> of their descendants. Over the past three centuries, that tension has
> been both soothed and deepened by the invention of whiteness and
> the resulting racialization of American culture.[1]

The pathology isn't that specific people or groups are evil. What
harms us all is the entrenched dynamics of domination (fight), division (flight), and indifference or dehumanization (freeze) that we've
each inherited from generations of trauma on all sides. Without seeing the root of our symptoms, we will continue to self-destruct as we
act out these dynamics again and again.

While choosing the simple narrative of good and evil is tempting,
we can't regain our humanity by dehumanizing others, even if those
people are the cause of our wounds. To rebuild our humanity, we must
restore it in everyone, not just those we deem good. We can't write off
the other as deplorable. Because all of us have internalized the dynamics
of perpetrator and victim, oppressor and oppressed, and us versus them.
And once this happens, we don't get to inhabit only one role in it.

As the Tibetan lama Druga Choegyal Rinpoche taught in the Shambhala Warrior Prophecy:

> This is not a battle between the good guys and the bad guys, but the line between good and evil runs through the landscape of every human heart.[2]

OWNING BOTH OUR DARKNESS AND OUR LIGHT

It's natural to want to only inhabit the light. So many of us have been fed stories of good conquering evil our entire lives. And yet my most profound growth has come from acknowledging and accepting the darkness living in me, just like everyone else.

On our first date, a past partner texted me a location to meet for a forest walk. But as I drove miles up an abandoned, overgrown gravel road to a dead end, my nervous system hollered an SOS as I realized that I forgot to even chat on the phone first to ensure that she was actually the gentle woman drinking tea on a mountaintop pictured in her dating profile.

Luckily, a playful tornado of a human jumped out of her car, and my body calmed as the rhythm of my heart shifted from a horror prelude to the high-pitched ballad of a tween yet to be jaded by love. I could be accused of intentionally getting us lost while we hiked, as I didn't want the thrill of so many grinning outbursts of "me too" of shared values and experiences to end.

We reminisced about that first date as we inhabited a blissful space for months.

But then we began to fight.

The more we fought, the more passionately we defended ourselves.

"I'm just so confused," I told my therapist, reaching for yet another tissue. "When we fight, I can't figure out who's the bad guy."

"The problem isn't who's the bad guy," my therapist responded. "It's that you're both so terrified of inhabiting this role that you get triggered the moment that you feel you're being accused of it, and then turn into it."

She was right. We had bonded over our shared passions and pain, both in our own lives and vicariously through our work with trauma survivors and social justice. And we both adapted to this hurt by choosing the role of the helper as a way of taking the side of the "good guy." But when the other showed us parts of ourselves that didn't match this ideal self-image, our shame alarms sounded, flipping us into fight mode to defend our goodness. But this defensive mode of mind loses its capacity to offer empathy and the slow, thoughtful "I statements" of nonviolent communication.[3]

"What if you hold all of these parts inside of you: good and bad," my therapist suggested. "What if rather than fighting to protect your goodness, you were allowed to acknowledge that messy trauma parts live in you, too, just like everyone else? Could you instead offer yourself the compassion of, 'I am this, too,' and invite it all to be here?"

A century ago, child psychoanalyst Melanie Klein identified how we split ourselves and others into all good or all bad—what she called the "good breast" and "bad breast"—especially when we're under stress. To a newcomer, the dialect of psychoanalysis sounds like a deadpan comedy. I spent years being supervised by psychoanalysts who would tell me that my patients saw me as a "toilet breast," while I responded with how castrated I felt, in the same tone I use to report a blood pressure. I suspect Sigmund Freud started the community off with so much phallic imagery that the women who followed must have felt a need to thrust some almighty breast symbols in there, too, and then it all got out of hand.

Klein fought with the theories of Freud and his daughter, Anna, to fracture the world of psychoanalysis into three groups, the Freudians, the Kleinians, and the Independents, who, like those observing our current political culture, were annoyed by the drama and division of both sides.

Freud believed we are motivated by sexual and aggressive drives, what he coined his *drive theory*, not a surprising assumption for a man who lived through two World Wars in a sexually repressed Victorian society. Klein, a mother of three, instead proposed that we're driven by our need to connect with others. She began studying mother-infant relationships, realizing that the quality of the connection between child and caregiver in the early years—not just the caregiver's ability to provide material needs such as food and shelter—deeply impacts how we regulate our nervous systems and relate to others in adult life. (In fact, they both succeeded in identifying some of our subcortical networks that drive our primary emotional experiences: lust, rage, care, and separation distress, once again proving the benefits of diverse perspectives.)

Klein explained that babies need their caregivers so desperately for love and survival that when they're nuzzled up at the symbolic breast, nurtured by someone who can tend to their emotional and physical needs, they experience the breast as all good. However, when babies are frustrated because their caregivers are absent or unable to hold their anxiety—perhaps their parent is busy with other children, work, or lost to their own stress response—they suddenly switch to believing the symbolic breast is all bad. If children have the privilege of experiencing somewhat consistent nurturing, what Klein's colleague, child psychiatrist Donald Winnicott, called the "good enough" caregiver, they learn that the good breast always comes back, and that the good breast and bad breast are one.

They realize that others are an integration of good and bad parts. Even when someone's frustrating them, they still have good parts, and even when someone is meeting their needs, they likely will frustrate them again. The same is true for themselves: they, too, have good and bad parts, just like everyone else. Klein named this acceptance of both good and bad in the same person the *depressive position*, because it's quite a downer to retire our fantasies of such shiny, ideal versions of ourselves and others. None of us are flawless superheroes.

Yet sometimes it's too painful to sit with this truth. The depressive position isn't a destination we arrive at and stay. Given enough stress, we circle back to splitting ourselves and others into all good or all bad in our stress response, especially if we haven't received consistent nurturing or safety early on to teach us to regulate our emotions and integrate the good and bad.[4] In essence, splitting is a defense that provides temporary respite. We hope to eventually return to a state of regulation in the depressive position if we are to face reality once the storm has passed. Authentic connection requires us to truly see each other in all our complexity: the light and dark live in us all.

THE INVISIBLE WOUNDS WE CARRY

It's deeply painful to acknowledge that darkness lives inside of us. Instead, so many of us choose to deny inequities, racism, supremacy, even genocides, rather than acknowledge how we participate in, perpetuate, benefit from, and internalize these systems. When we refuse to see the darkness that we carry from our pasts, we risk acting it out, again and again.

Historical trauma accumulates in subsequent generations when our ancestors didn't have the opportunity to heal from it.[5] That's why it's so important for us to make it conscious—see our reactions as embodiments of trauma—and reintegrate it into our whole understanding of ourselves and our world. Every generation that works toward healing the trauma living in their own bodies helps to slow its transmission to the next one.

Yet so much of trauma is hidden in our cells, without the scars to tell the story of how it got there. We often think of the effects of direct violence when we speak of trauma, the physical harm caused at the hands of another. Psychiatry's *DSM* falls into this trap, limiting a formal diagnosis of post-traumatic stress disorder (PTSD) to only those who have "exposure to actual or threatened death, serious injury, or sexual violence." But as a trauma therapist myself, physical harm is not what my patients identify as having the most enduring impact: it's the emotional wounds from interpersonal trauma. And not only do injuries inflicted by specific people harm us, but also our relationships to the larger communities and systems around us, especially the bystanders who allow violence to continue without seeing and standing up for those who are being harmed. So much of the time, trauma results from inaction, when individuals, communities, or societal systems deny or neglect our fundamental rights, needs, and dignity.

After witnessing the Nazis arrest his father as a child during Germany's occupation of Norway in World War II, Norwegian sociologist Johan Galtung dedicated his life to studying peace and equity, creating the Peace Research Institute Oslo. Galtung expanded our concept of violence beyond the direct violence of one person injuring another. He identified structural violence as causing a more insidious yet significant kind of trauma. Having witnessed the harms of poverty, Galtung recognized that no one person was to blame; the cause lay with the injustices embedded within the collective structure of society. He also identified cultural violence to describe how our societies shape us to dehumanize the "other" with indifference, allowing us to perpetuate violence without recognizing the inhumanity of our actions.

SURVIVAL OF THE NURTURED

One of Galtung's students, Otto Scharmer, identified another source of trauma that often lies hidden in the shadows of everyday experience, what he defines as *attentional violence*, of not being seen by others. This attentional violence explains the trauma we experience in the face of injuries from our attachment to caregivers.

We already touched upon how the sensitivity of children's alarm systems adapt to their caregiver's capacity to connect with them. If children's caregivers are always preoccupied with safety or securing food, housing, and other basic needs rather than attending to their children's emotional needs—or are simply not around, the children adapt by dismissing the need for attachment with others to help them survive in this tough world. They disavow their basic need to connect with others, both avoiding (flight) or rejecting (fight) intimacy as adults or defending against the desire with denial and numbness (a freeze response).

But if children get a taste of the rewards of the attentiveness of their caregivers, though only intermittently, they adapt by fixating on their precarious connections with others, always anxious that others will leave. To get the other's attention, they learn to be more pleasing, engaging in their fawn response. If that doesn't work, they move into their fight response in desperate attempts to demand the other's attention.

Sometimes, a child's caregiver is attentive in one moment, then harmful in another. This leads to a *disorganized* attachment strategy, where the child is both drawn to a caregiver for support, but also fears them, so they swing between moving toward and moving away from their caregiver(s). In this situation, children try all their defenses: fawn, fight, flight, and freeze, in a confusing dance of conflicting needs—both to be cared for and safe from harm.

However, if a child's caregiver appears mostly calm, connected, and capable, able to somewhat consistently respond to their emotional needs much of the time—remember a caregiver only needs to be "good enough" at showing up—then they, too, get the privilege of feeling confident in their capacity to regulate their own nervous systems and relate securely to others. This is because we learn how to self-soothe and regulate our emotions (known as *self-regulation*) through repeated and consistent acts of *co-regulation* from caregivers.

Children are volcanos of emotional dysregulation, as our upstairs brain (the prefrontal cortex) doesn't complete its development until we're twenty-four years old. They need to dump their mess of overwhelming emotions into the bodies and minds of their caregiver, who receives it, makes sense of it, and then relays it back in a more tolerable form (for example, *Oh sweetie, it makes so much sense you're upset! You're so mad at your sister when she pushes you, and you need her to know that it's not okay to touch you that way*).

When children don't receive this from others, they don't have the privilege of learning self-regulation and can struggle with emotional dysregulation as an adult, fluctuating between unbearable emotions and rigid defenses to fawn, fight, flee, and numb out the distress. Luckily, we can always learn this skill later in life. When we engage with people who consistently attune to our emotional experiences—either in therapy or in healthy relationships in our day-to-day lives—we learn to more easily regulate our emotions as adults, although it takes time to unlearn old attachment strategies. In this way, we can learn to trust and relate securely to others even if we missed this opportunity as a child.

The attachment strategies that we adopt—whether secure, avoidant, anxious, or disorganized—don't reflect how "good" or "bad" our caregivers are as humans. We are privileged with secure attachment early on when our caregiver(s) and their ancestors had the opportunity of living in secure-enough environments that could meet their physical and emotional needs, or had enough access to it later in life. To be able to hold and process a child's eruptions of emotion, the caregiver needs to have had the opportunity to learn self-regulation themselves.

This is where intergenerational learning and trauma come in. If the caregiver's own nervous system is overactivated or shut down from their own stress reactions, they don't have the capacity to co-regulate their child. It's not that they don't want to; they simply can't offer that support. If caregivers have never been nurtured themselves in this way, despite desiring to give everything to their child, they can't offer what they've never received. In this way, trauma moves seamlessly through the generations, invisible to its owners, yet deeply impacting every cell of their bodies through inflammation and dysregulation.

It's so tempting to blame our parents when we acknowledge how persistently our past relationships affect our present. The most important nuance I've learned, in both my own therapy as a mom and daughter and as a therapist and supervisor to others, is to both acknowledge how our past relationships (especially within our family of origin) profoundly impact our mental health *and* to see how our caregiver(s) lacked the capacity to be more attentive and helpful because of their own adaptations to stress and trauma. I've learned to hold compassion and empathy for everyone. We can also apply this compassion to ourselves as caregivers when we feel like our own struggles have impacted our kids. Which brings us back to that uncomfortable depressive position again, grieving that despite our own and others' good intentions, we're all connected, so the trauma and hardship we've all faced affect each other.

I'm careful to stay away from blaming caregivers when I present the last two decades of scientific studies strongly linking adverse childhood experiences (ACEs) to illness, as we discussed in Chapter Three. We must instead understand the structural violence and historical trauma underlying these experiences. In this way, Matt Burkey, a Canadian child psychiatrist trained in public health from Johns Hopkins University, advocates for preventing ACEs through a population lens. He asks, "What are the underlying upstream factors like poverty, inequality and education that are leading to such high rates of abuse, neglect and other adversities?" Instead of blaming the caregivers of people with high ACE scores, we need to see them also as survivors of the inequitable systems and historical trauma that harms their children's health, not the cause of it.

This is where transformational justice comes in. We can't just see those who perpetrate violence as an isolated source of the problem. The pathology is our dynamics of dominance, division, and dehumanization passing through the generations of our interdependent collective that keep harming us all. We can notice when these dynamics are playing out in our relationships between individuals, groups, nations, and the environment because our safety and security feel under threat. Then, through the skills we are introducing in the next chapters, we can work to regulate all of our systems back to the balanced state capable of empathy, cooperation, and co-regulation.

If we all dysregulate into these entrenched dynamics, then our stress reactions become our permanent culture that indoctrinates each generation. We regress to adopting cultures of extreme individualism

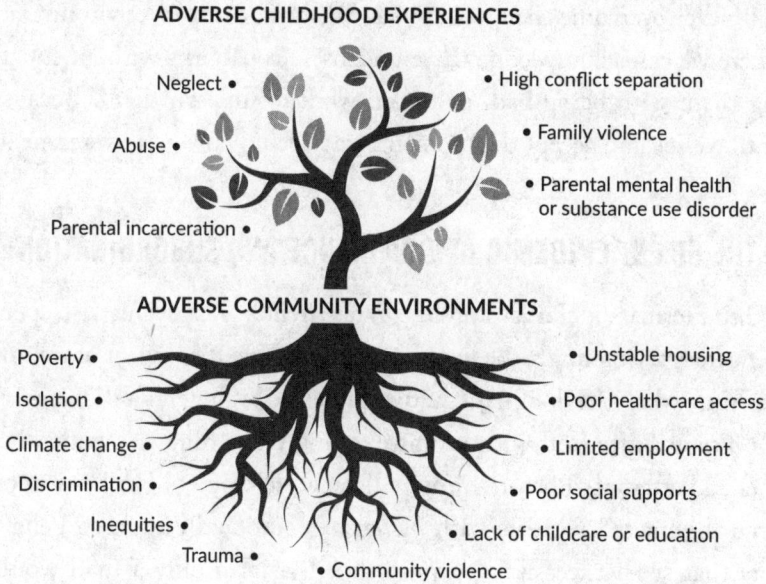

ADVERSE CHILDHOOD EXPERIENCES

Neglect •   • High conflict separation

Abuse •   • Family violence

                                             • Parental mental health
Parental incarceration •   or substance use disorder

ADVERSE COMMUNITY ENVIRONMENTS

Poverty •   • Unstable housing

Isolation •   • Poor health-care access

Climate change •   • Limited employment

Discrimination •   • Poor social supports

Inequities •   • Lack of childcare or education

Trauma •
              • Community violence

Adverse Community Environments are to blame for ACEs, not caregivers.
Adapted from Iles et al. (2022).

that disregard our interdependence with each other, or extreme forms of collectivism that discriminate against our differences. Or we may spend so long stuck in our fawn, fight, flight, or freeze responses that it feels as if we become them, our identities reduced to either perpetrator or victim.

For this reason, many decolonized healing programs refuse to use terms like *perpetrator* and *victim*, preferring instead *people who have caused harm* and *people who have been harmed*.[6] When someone acts in ways that are harmful, they are not seen as a criminal in need of punishment, but a person in need of teaching and healing from their community.[7] Approaching justice in this way does not take away from the need to exercise accountability, regulations, consequences, and boundaries to prevent the person who caused harm from harming again. Both can be practiced at the same time.

Until we see and accept how we've all been socialized to internalize these disordered dynamics that so easily get enacted with stress, we will never overcome their hold on us. We need to create environments where we can acknowledge these unconscious patterns without equating them with being bad, and then work to unlearn them. Because until we see and accept the problem, we have no power to overcome it.

THE SILENT EPIDEMIC OF DOMINANCE AND SUBORDINATION

Judith Herman, a Harvard professor, researcher, and psychiatrist, spent her career trying to get the world to acknowledge the impact of trauma at a time when the dominant culture preferred to pretend it didn't exist.

Freud started off with promise, doing something few male doctors had attempted before him: he listened to women. For hour upon hour, he invited patients with *hysteria*—emotionally charged behaviors that seem excessive or dysregulated (a term only a man would choose to name after the uterus)—to lie on his velvet couch and *free associate*, sharing with him everything that entered their minds.

What he heard was a lot of trauma, especially the sexual exploitation of women and children. So, as a scientifically trained neurologist, he published his findings in 1896, entitled *The Aetiology of Hysteria*. He diagnosed the cause of hysteria as early childhood sexual trauma, defining this finding as the *caput Nili*—the source of the Nile—of neuropathology.

However, because Freud's clientele were the elites of the dominant culture of Victorian society—the same circles with whom he puffed cigars and holidayed in the Alps—he received a lot of pushback from accusing the families of his "well-bred" peers of sexual abuse. Rather than face the discomfort of the correct diagnosis—that the dynamics of dominance inherited from many generations before them were infecting their own families—Freud chose to cover up his findings.

He stopped believing his patients, suggesting the memories were not real, but simply their fantasies, setting the stage for Western society to deny and disregard the violence that so many people repeatedly faced for the next hundred years. It took until 1980 to legitimize trauma when a social movement of Vietnam veterans fought to validate the diagnosis of PTSD. "It was much easier for people to recognize trauma in war veterans, because you couldn't deny that they'd been to war," Herman told me. "Whereas in the so-called private sphere of the abuse of women and children, often there were no witnesses outside the family."

Herman argued that trauma was not simply a rare affliction affecting war veterans but an injury too commonly experienced by people exposed to oppression, abuse, and sexual violence in their everyday lives. "Trauma is trauma," she explained. "The concepts I'm describing about trauma apply to the violence of dominance and subordination, whether that's based on gender, race, class, or religion."

Herman defines trauma as a social illness—the violence of dominance and subordination—that requires a social cure. We need to collectively bring it to light to heal the injuries that people who've experienced harm typically carry alone.

But so many of us bystanders would prefer to keep these dark parts of humanity hidden, because they're too disturbing to bear. "It's hard to talk about trauma if you don't have a social movement that names the problem, because the bystanders and the wider community would just as soon not think about it," Herman told me. We often choose our own comfort by turning away instead of sharing in the pain of humanity's cruelty and injustices with those who experience trauma, especially when we're benefiting from the power imbalances and inequities that fueled the harm.

Denying that a person responsible for sexual or family violence is capable of dominating and exploiting women and children because he's a "nice guy," that supremacy and inequities exist at all, or that our privilege comes at the cost of colonialism and systemic oppression is easier than accepting trauma's painful truths. And it's more comfortable to blame those who've been harmed—"she was asking for it," "immigrants are poisoning the blood of our country," or "people live in poverty because of laziness or lack of merit." For this reason, civil rights and anti-war movements, #MeToo, Every Child Matters, and

Black Lives Matter, play vital roles in healing the fragments of our traumas that hide in plain sight. We need to share the role of holding the pain with those who've been harmed by acknowledging that this darkness lives within our communities, our world, and ourselves.

"I was taught that keeping quiet kept the peace, until I realized whose peace it's keeping," said gender-based violence expert and psychologist Thema Bryant in her TEDx talk, "You Can Heal Intergenerational Trauma." "The offenders are at peace. The people who don't want to deal with it are at peace." Instead, when people who've experienced harm receive acknowledgment, accountability, and repair from their communities, their sense of belonging—and faith in humanity—is restored, she explained. And so is the bystanders'.

STAGE ONE OF HEALING: SEEKING SAFETY

Herman describes four stages of trauma recovery that have been widely adopted across therapy approaches. The first is to establish safety and stability. We cannot heal from our past if our present continues to be dangerous, persistently overwhelming our nervous systems. We need to seek safety both in our outer worlds and in our ability to feel safe in our own bodies, minds, and souls.

As we explored in the last chapter, to reestablish a sense of safety, we can work together to decrease everyone's exposure to unsafe environments (such as collaborating to help change our harmful systems or set boundaries with those causing harm). Even when that's not possible, we can still increase our sense of inner safety by anchoring in the ABCs, with establishing agency, bonding, and containment. In the next chapters, we will learn many other skills to help regulate our nervous systems and emotional alarms to feel more safety within our bodies and minds.

We often think of safety as freedom from fear. But Herman describes trauma as a condition not only of fear, but of shame. "It shakes your trust in people," she told me. "It affects your sense of self, your sense of relationships, and sense of safety in the world." When a stressful event is impersonal, such as an earthquake, then we develop a heightened fear alarm to ensure we don't miss the next physically threatening event. But when people harm us, shame is the more common alarm.

As we discussed in Chapter One, our shame alarms warn us that it's not safe for others to hold our vulnerable parts, that they may reject or harm us if we show ourselves fully. When we experience interpersonal harm, we adapt by making our shame alarm more sensitive—we monitor others for the slightest sign of rejection or armor ourselves by hiding any potential vulnerabilities that could be unsafe in the hands of others.

Brené Brown defines shame as the intensely painful experience of believing that we are flawed and therefore unworthy of love, belonging, and connection. This definition shows the impact of our evolutionary shame alarm when our thinking minds get a hold of it. We concoct the story that we are the problem rather than see that its intended purpose is to alert us to situations where others may be rejecting or unsafe. But shame has nothing to do with our actual worthiness. It reflects how safe those around us are, or have been in the past.

Our minds often take this shame signal and displace the blame onto ourselves. We have more agency if we're the problem, because then it's within our control to fix. Blaming ourselves can feel more empowering than acknowledging that the people we depend on for survival and belonging are unsafe. This is how interpersonal harm leads to Brown's definition of shame. When we're powerless to prevent threats to our belonging, our adaptive brains convince us that we're the problem in order to maintain a sense of agency. This defense creates a false narrative, but it keeps away the anguish of losing faith in those we depend on to survive, and in humanity itself.

Recovering from trauma, therefore, requires healing the wider communities and systems around us. We need to restore our belief in the safety of others and our belonging in just communities. Only then can our screaming alarms silence. When others meet our vulnerable parts with safety and acceptance, we can learn that nothing is inherently wrong with us. In the same way, we can stop projecting the blame onto people we've divided ourselves from and instead see their vulnerable parts and humanity, too.

STAGE TWO OF HEALING: REMEMBRANCE AND MOURNING

"I suddenly feel horrible," my patients commonly share with me. "I don't understand. I just can't stop crying out of nowhere."

They continue to tell me that it doesn't seem to make any sense. They've just overcome a major stressor, such as leaving a toxic environment or relationship, or completing a court case or round of chemo, or maybe they've finally found a supportive partner or community, secured housing, or taken time off.

"That's wonderful," I tell them. "It means you're finally safe enough to feel."

"Well, I preferred being numb," they usually respond, yet with a smile of relief.

I get it; my nervous system's been trained to jump into the subtle numbness of freeze the moment I can't find my car keys. I'm more comfortable in a crisis, when I don't have any pesky emotions to entertain. But we can't run from our feelings forever. Well, we can, but the cost of suppressing them is a constant stress response that leads to chronic inflammation, emotional emptiness, and painful symptoms, so it's not an approach I'd recommend. Trust me, I've tried it.

We must feel safe and regulated in the present before we can revisit the past. It's a slow, integrative process, Herman told me, "where you grieve and make meaning of what happened and transform your traumatic memory into a narrative memory that is part of your life story but not your whole life story."

Rather than having undigested trauma fragments involuntarily taking over the reins of our bodies and minds when triggered in our day-to-day life, we invite the trauma memories into our awareness and learn to hold them with safety and agency, all while being supported by others (fulfilling the ABCs of regulation). In this way, we reintegrate our fragments of trauma back into our life story so that the trauma memories are stored in the same predictable way as our nontraumatic memories.

There is no single way to do this work, since each of us is grounded in our own temperaments, cultures, and communities, influencing how we best match our healing to our own lived experiences and lineages. Sometimes, it's done in words, music, or art, or it can be processed in the body, through meditation or cultural or religious ceremony. Sometimes, we process with a therapist, or we may choose to do so in community.

I was fortunate to witness the premiere of the Cambodian opera *Where Elephants Weep* in the nation's capital, Phnom Penh, because one of my best friends was in the cast. Commissioned by the Cambodian Living Arts, the show was inspired by the life of its founder, genocide survivor and refugee Arn Chorn-Pond. When Pol Pot's Khmer Rouge took power in 1975, killing over two million civilians in the following four years, they sent nine-year-old Chorn-Pond to a prison camp with hundreds of other children.

"I was in a temple where they killed three or four times a day," he said.[8] "They told us to watch and not show any emotion at all. They would kill us if we reacted . . . if we showed that we cared about the victims. So, I had to shut it all off . . . I made myself numb." He was then forced to fight on the front lines as a child soldier and witnessed children killed right next to him for disobeying orders.

"Those who lived under the brutal armed regime of the Khmer Rouge could not stand up against them by demonstrating or expressing themselves in public," explained the opera's composer, Him Sophy, who also survived the Killing Fields.[9] Sophy and Chorn-Pond hoped to empower their fellow Cambodians to regain the capacity to express themselves once again, to put words to their shared history, to feel the emotions together, and thus heal their collective trauma.

In a similar way, social worker Maria Yellow Horse Brave Heart describes a model of processing the cumulative trauma and unresolved grief that her community endures from colonization.[10] By the time my ancestors fled Russia to North Dakota, the land's original stewards, the Lakota people, had endured genocide, forced relocations, broken treaties, the prohibition of cultural practices, and continued systemic oppression at the hands of settlers like my ancestors. In Brave Heart's approach, community members first stimulate memories of historical trauma and educate each other about the lasting impacts of colonization. Then they create space for group sharing while modeling how to stay balanced together as they hold such painful emotions, all while grounding in their traditional culture, rituals, and communal support.

Tamika Middleton and Cara Page founded the Kindred Southern Healing Justice Collective to respond to the collective trauma, grief, burnout, and violence that their community organizers were holding. They come together to elevate their own cultural and spiritual practices of the American South to create ritual and sacred spaces for grief, loss, and reflection. Middleton and Page hope to transform trauma collectively with healing strategies rooted in place and ancestry, recognizing that no single model of care is sufficient for everyone. Instead, they center care on choice, consent, and the ability to determine how and what healing looks like for each person as part of their own community and ancestry.

STAGES THREE AND FOUR OF HEALING: RECONNECTION AND SOCIAL JUSTICE

The third stage of recovery from trauma involves reconnecting with our community in the present, "to imagine things you can do and be and become that you couldn't imagine before," Herman explained. Rather than get stuck reliving our unprocessed past, we can move forward to live to our full potential in the present.

This links with the final stage of social justice: to rebuild a moral community that acknowledges the harm, supports the people who have experienced it, and prevents it from happening again. "If trauma is truly a social problem, and indeed it is, then recovery cannot simply be a private, individual matter," argued Herman. If trauma results from being disempowered, then empowerment must be a central principle of recovery; if trauma shames and isolates, then recovery must take place in community.

When Herman researched what people with trauma needed to heal, they envisioned justice as healing the damaged relationships with the bystanders in their communities. "The number one requirement was public acknowledgment of the harm," she said. "They weren't that focused on the offender. They were much more focused on the bystanders, because trauma isolates people and shames them. They wanted to regain the respect and validation from the communities or their family. When the community embraces the survivor, justice is served."

The betrayal of the broader community, Herman's research showed, "the actions or inactions of bystanders—all those who are complicit in or who prefer not to know about the abuse or who blame the victims," often cause deeper wounds than those inflicted directly by the people perpetrating the violence. The betrayal can be from an individual bystander not speaking up against abuse, institutions not believing or supporting those who have been harmed, or the entire world failing to stop a genocide. As Martin Luther King Jr. said, "In the end, we will remember not the words of our enemies, but the silence of our friends."

Speaking up against the dynamics of domination, division, and dehumanization that infects members of our collective requires courage, especially when those committing grave harm are allies, leaders, relatives, or people who have been harmed by trauma and discrimination themselves. It's why so many bystanders around the world remain silent in the face of crimes against humanity.

"These wounds are part of the social ecology of violence, in which crimes against subordinated and marginalized people are rationalized, tolerated, and rendered invisible," Herman explained. Instead, justice involves being part of a community where everyone belongs, everyone's human rights are respected, and everyone has a voice.

Patricia Vickers, of the Tsimshian and Heiltsuk nations, studied ancestral law and healing through Indigenous cultural teachings and ceremony for her PhD. "When there's harm done, there's a spiritual imbalance. And how balance is restored is with a process," she told me. Their process includes those who perpetrated the harm acknowledging what they did wrong. Then the people who were harmed share what harm was done, and the person who caused the harm listens and acknowledges that they see the damage. Finally, the person who caused the harm owns what they did in front of the community. "These are the things that are missing in our society today," Vickers explains. "If you have no way of making it right, what you have is this state of imbalance."

This process echoes the Truth and Reconciliation Commission, chosen by South Africa's first democratically elected cabinet, the Government of National Unity (GNU), led by Nelson Mandela. The GNU departed from the country's past atrocities of the white supremacy of apartheid with aims of sharing power and building peace among its fractured groups. Rather than seizing the power that was so horrifically stolen from Black South Africans and continuing the dynamics of dominance, division, and dehumanization, but in reverse roles, the new unity government forged a different path, choosing reparations over revenge and peace over power.

The coalition government created the Truth and Reconciliation Commission (TRC) to address the severe human rights violations spanning from 1960 to 1994 during apartheid as "a necessary exercise to enable South Africans to come to terms with their past on a morally accepted basis and to advance the cause of reconciliation."[11] Archbishop and human rights activist Desmond Tutu chaired the Commission with the interconnected spirit of Ubuntu. If social harmony and solidarity creates the greatest good for us, Tutu explained, then we heal from crimes against humanity by reestablishing harmonious relationships between those who both caused and suffered the harms.[12]

The Commission listened to twenty-one thousand people who perpetrated, experienced, and witnessed the harms of apartheid—two thousand of whom shared in public sessions. It acted to record and bear witness to the human rights abuses of apartheid, provide rehabilitation and reparations to those harmed, and grant amnesty from civil and criminal prosecution to some of the people who perpetrated harm. The hearings did not have a blanket policy of amnesty; they evaluated every person's case to assess the need for additional prosecution.[13] "The envisioned overall function of all recommendations is to ensure non-repetition, healing, and healthy co-existence," explained South Africa's Ministry of Justice.[14]

The Commission also created a register of reconciliation to provide opportunities for bystanders to express their regrets and remorse for failing to prevent human rights violations. "The register has been established in response to a deep wish for reconciliation in the hearts of many South Africans—people who did not perhaps commit gross violations of human rights but nevertheless wish to indicate their regret for failures in the past to do all they could have done to prevent such violations; people who want to demonstrate in some symbolic way their commitment to a new kind of future in which human rights abuses will not take place," explained TRC commissioner Mary Burton.

While the TRC helped to mend South Africa's moral community, the process alone couldn't achieve all the goals of justice, healing, and repair. One of the biggest criticisms of the TRC is how it focused only on the accountability of individuals while failing to disrupt the foundation of the atrocities: the ongoing structural inequities and power imbalances that maintained the socio-economic order of apartheid.[15]

Medicine has grappled with similar challenges when approaching medical errors, the third leading cause of patient deaths in the US and Canada.[16] We can't only focus on the individuals making mistakes without exploring the systemic issues that drive them. A large global review showed that health-care professionals in work cultures with the most hierarchies, power imbalances, and demands for conformity and obedience speak up the least when they notice a safety concern.[17] Conversely, medical errors were reduced when health-care systems promoted inclusive cultures of psychological safety that respected their staff's diverse views and allowed them to contribute new ideas, acknowledge errors, and challenge the system. When health-care teams gather in nonpunitive M&M (Morbidity and Mortality) rounds to explore what went wrong at all levels of the system, we are more capable of supporting all parties by working together to identify and acknowledge individual and systemic problems, repair the harms, and fix the underlying structures to prevent it from happening again.

Compassionately acknowledging that we all make mistakes, that our stress responses can cause dysregulated behaviors that harm, and that systemic problems underlie many of our individual actions doesn't disregard the vital need for regulations, accountability, consequences, and boundaries, especially when those who are perpetuating harm fail to stop their violence. We must also take a clear stance on what behavior is not permitted in our moral community.

Now, more than ever, we need to identify when both our collective's individuals and its larger systems have regressed to the dynamics of domination, division, and dehumanization, so we can fairly and firmly protect our human rights and safety. We can only heal the imbalances in our systems when our culture values justice, with the appropriate governance in place to prevent harm.

We can both practice empathy and compassion for each other's challenges and, also, protect ourselves from ongoing harm.

TENDING TO OUR WOUNDS

Not everything that is faced can be changed, but
nothing can be changed until it's faced.

—JAMES BALDWIN

So where do we begin when facing the specific traumas living in our individual bodies? I like to start by validating that all our inner experiences make sense, even if these intense reactions seem irrational at times. Sometimes, rather than the alarm matching the danger of the present situation, it's recognizing patterns of danger learned from our past or that of our ancestors' trauma.

"If something is hysterical, then it is usually historical," Resmaa Menakem teaches in *My Grandmother's Hands*. "If your (or anyone's reaction) to a current situation has more (or far less) energy than it normally would, then it likely involves energy from ancient historical trauma that has lost its context. In the present, your body is experiencing unmetabolized trauma from the past."

The key to working with the intergenerational wisdom that lives in our bodies is in learning to decipher what's a useful alarm for our present situation and what's a historical—and at times misleading—alarm, carried in our bodies as an adaptation to recognize risky patterns from past dangers. Historical alarms may or may not be helpful today, since they operate (often unconsciously) on autopilot, offering the past's solutions to today's problems.

In the next chapters, we will explore how to bring a kind attention to these alarms so we can both hear their important messages and assess whether they indicate a present danger or a false alarm from a system sensitized by past threats. Then we will learn skills to offer ourselves and others compassion, understanding that even our messiest moments make sense when we see them through this lens of adaptations to our past environments.

Maybe extending compassion to a child whose dysregulation shows up as disruptive behavior is easier for us because we can clearly see the innocence of their stress responses. Can we offer the same compassion to ourselves and the adults around us whose so-called bad behavior we villainize? Rather than dehumanizing ourselves and others with blame and shame, can we see that our personal or historical trauma often steers our behaviors into ugly places simply to survive?

FIVE

HOW TO BE AN
ANTI-ASSHOLE

One does not become enlightened by imagining figures
of light, but by making the darkness conscious. The latter
procedure, however, is disagreeable and therefore not popular.

—C. G. Jung

"IT'S JUST THAT YOU HAVE TO MAKE SURE THAT THE READER ACTUALLY LIKES YOUR PRO-
tagonist," a classmate offered as we workshopped my creative writing.
"Your protagonist sounds a bit like an asshole."

A surge of shame suddenly short-circuited my capacity to make
constructive use of her feedback. Having repeatedly made the mistake
of reading the online comments section about my writing as a journalist, I can usually swallow many shots of critical feedback without
a flush. But I had just shared my memoir writing for the first time, a
sober game of strip poker where I'd let the readers see the naked mess
in my head. And now I feared that my classmate had finally discovered my secret, that I am, in fact, an asshole.

All week I checked in with friends and family: "Do you think I'm
an asshole?"

Everyone stamped me with the approval of not being an asshole.
But each reassurance provided only momentary relief.

Then one friend changed the narrative.

"So what if you can act like an asshole sometimes?" she asked, with a playful grin.

"You're right, I can be an asshole."

"Can't we all?"

When I talk about being an asshole, I mean that we all have ugly thoughts, feelings, urges, and body sensations that we don't really like, let alone want others to know about. We don't have much control over the experiences that arise within us, especially the ones that automatically pop into our minds and bodies. What we can do is learn to relate more gently to them, rather than fight an endless battle to deny, judge, or banish them out of existence.

I titled this chapter "*How to Be an Anti-Asshole*" in deep appreciation of the teachings of Ibram X. Kendi, the director of the Center for Antiracist Research at Boston University, who titled his bible of a book *How to Be an Antiracist*.[1] We all have racist parts, just like we have asshole ones. We've all internalized unconscious biases, beliefs, and reactions from the cultures and environments we've inhabited, including the dynamics of dominance, division, and indifference. And we all have nervous systems that involuntarily punt us into fight, flight, or freeze the moment we feel threatened. Of course, we all react in ways we don't like. But denying the reality of our hardwiring and socialization doesn't help us live in line with our values.

Let me be clear: I'm not suggesting that you go around acting like an asshole. But the first step to acting in healthy ways is to recognize what's already here without judging ourselves for experiencing it. Shame and blame drive our messy parts back into hiding, so we lose access to the inner awareness that allows us to learn and grow.

Let's take racism, for example. "Denial is the heartbeat of racism, beating across ideologies, races, and nations," Kendi says. "The only way to undo racism is to consistently identify and describe it—and then dismantle it." Despite focusing his career on antiracism and being Black himself, Kendi accepts that, growing up in a racist country, he, too, has internalized racist beliefs and subscribed to racist policies just like the rest of us. But rather than preaching the delusion that these biases don't exist, he supports being "antiracist," to acknowledge these racist practices and beliefs and then intentionally replace them with ones that promote equality.

One of the obstacles to disclosing our biases honestly, says anti-racism educator Robin DiAngelo, is the moral "good/bad binary" attached, what she describes as "a character flaw assassination."[2] DiAngelo tries to disarm her audiences by changing the narrative from "You are racist and only bad people are racist," which leads to shame, defensiveness, and shutting down, to "Racism is a system into which we are all socialized," which allows us to feel safe enough to acknowledge our biases, receive constructive feedback, and change.

"We consider a challenge to our racial worldviews as a challenge to our very identities as good, moral people," she explains. Instead, we must accept that we all have racist—and asshole—thoughts, feelings, and urges to act as an inevitable consequence of internalizing the world's intergenerational dynamics of domination, division, and dehumaniza-tion. Rather than feel offended or shamed when they are pointed out, we could express gratitude, because the awareness empowers us to grow and change. It's the same with all the other ugly and painful thoughts, feelings, and urges inside us. This gentle, safe noticing of all our inner experiences creates the freedom to choose healthier responses.

While we can't control our knee-jerk thoughts, feelings, and reac-tions, if we notice them, we can influence the next ones. But so many of us have never been granted the opportunity to learn to pay atten-tion to what's happening within us.

Awareness of our inner experiences—our thoughts, feelings, body sensations, and urges to act—is the foundation of all the other skills to manage our mental health. Yet rather than admit that we're all talk-ing about the same thing, experts often pretend that they've uniquely discovered a new phenomenon, from observing ego to self-observation, labeling, decentering, reflective functioning, mentalization, witnessing, metacognition, and mindfulness. I'm not going to pick a team by choosing a favorite term, because I've learned from many and it's all the same stuff. The consensus, though, is that it's not just what we're doing—paying attention—that matters, but *how* we're doing it: we learn to observe our experiences with kindness, curiosity, and acceptance.

When I teach mindfulness classes, I sometimes have participants return after the first session feeling worse, with them judging themselves for having "bad" thoughts, feelings, or urges. So, before we learn to practice attention, we need to ensure that we first notice these old habits of judging ourselves and meet our thoughts and feelings with compassion. Because if you can't pay attention kindly, it's better to not pay attention at all.

THE SIMPLE POWER OF NOTICING

We tend to think of meditation in only one
way. But life itself is a meditation.
—RAUL JULIA

When offering mindfulness meditations, I invite participants to focus on an anchor (such as the breath, body, or sound) and then be curious about the thoughts, body sensations, emotions, and action urges that inevitably arise in our awareness as part of being a healthy human being. The goal of mindfulness meditation is not to have an empty or nondistracted mind, but to learn to relate kindly to the millions of messy experiences that automatically enter our awareness.

Formal meditation is like exercising at the gym. Just as we strengthen our bodies so they can function better in our day-to-day lives, we practice mindfulness to strengthen our brains so we're more able to offer this kind attention whenever we need it. And as with physical fitness, where we can strengthen our bodies in a variety of informal ways, from dancing to cleaning, we can practice mindfulness informally by simply paying attention with kindness to any moment in the day.

When facilitating dialectical behavior therapy (DBT) or cognitive behavioral therapy (CBT) groups, I instruct participants to bring awareness to their inner worlds by labeling their thoughts, feelings, body sensations, and action urges. When I provide mentalization, psychodynamic, interpersonal, and so many of the other therapies we're trained in as psychiatrists, I guide my patients to practice noticing their emotions, thoughts, body sensations, and urges and how they relate to their present or past interpersonal situations. This same technique exists in so many other styles of therapy.

The foundation for almost every therapy or mental health skill is to build awareness of our inner experiences. Bringing awareness to our thoughts, feelings, body sensations, and urges redirects our brain from its fast, instinctive, emotional limbic system to the slower, intentional, and empathic prefrontal cortex. Many studies show that labeling our inner experiences activates areas in our prefrontal cortex that reduce our limbic brain's firing, dampening the intensity of our negative emotions and reactivity.[3] Bringing awareness to our inner experiences in this way is known as a *top-down* strategy, where we regulate our brains and bodies from the higher brain center, the prefrontal cortex. (In later chapters, we will cover the equally important *bottom-up* approaches to regulating our brains through our bodies.)

THE MOUNTAIN AND THE WEATHER

I often invite people to imagine themselves as a mountain—their observing self—solid and unmoving, witnessing all sorts of seasons on their surface.[4]

In the same way, we can notice all the changing weather patterns in our own lives—our passing thoughts, feelings, urges to act, and body sensations, as well as the storms in our outer worlds—while staying grounded in this observing self. We watch it all arise and pass, again and again, with an attitude of kindness and compassion. Whether we're in a shame wave or overtaken with a flood of rage or grief, it can feel as if we are the weather. But all these inner experiences arise and pass, too, if we don't make them worse by pushing them away or get stuck spinning in thoughts about them.

"How we are isn't who we are," Zen Reverend angel Kyodo williams taught me during a radical dharma conversations retreat on racial healing. How we're feeling in any one moment, even when we're activated into our most asshole-like defenses, doesn't define who we are. And who we are is the one who's able to observe and hold all of the constantly changing experiences that pass through us every day. When we observe these changing events both within and outside of us with a kind and curious awareness, we become the mountain with room to hold it all.

As we notice storms arising within us, we can label the thoughts, feelings, action urges, and body sensations as passing weather systems, staying grounded in our awareness practice of the observing mountain. We can say to ourselves, *Ah, there's a shame alarm/a worry thought/an urge to fight*, and kindly observe it, giving us a moment to pause and respond in line with our values, rather than reacting habitually in old patterns of autopilot. If we feel that we're getting pulled into the storm on the surface of our mountain, we can lean into the solid base of our mountain, anchoring ourselves into the ground by noticing the sensations of our feet or body on the floor.

STEPPING OUT OF AUTOPILOT

We often want our brain to stay in cruise control to be efficient and restful. For much of the time, whether we're breathing, commuting, or showering, autopilot saves us energy so our minds can focus on other things. We would be utterly exhausted if we had to be fully attentive to everything all the time.

The problem with autopilot is that it can't adapt to new obstacles in the road ahead. Autopilot applies past solutions to today's problem. Yet new and complex situations often bring unique challenges that require

a fresh lens of attention. We can rest in autopilot when yesterday's solution works just fine. But we can also learn to step out of autopilot to
bring a more careful attention to situations that require new responses.

Remember how we're wired for connection and attachment to others to ensure our survival? Many of us have learned patterns of relating to people to help us survive in the past groups of our lives, such as
our families, peer groups, workplace cultures, and wider communities.
Someone asks, "How are you?" and our culture may have conditioned
us to answer, "Fine," before we even have time to reflect on whether this
response is true or helpful.

We often adopt automatic patterns—what we call *implicit learning*,
because it's outside of our awareness—that served us well in past environments but may no longer be helpful today. I learned from a young
age that my membership in the many groups of my life seemed secured
by performing, pleasing, and appeasing everyone, at the cost of supress-
ing my own authenticity and needs. Over time, this pattern pushed me
into symptoms of anxiety and low mood—and probably a lot of chronic
inflammation—sending me a warning that my autopilot was no longer
helpful.

I needed to get out of cruise control and drive manually so I could
better understand the nuances of how I was living my life in ways that
were hurting me. I learned from paying attention to resentment and
fear where I needed to set healthier boundaries in relationships. Low
mood and grief showed me where I needed to refocus my energy and
what hard changes I could make so my life would feel more rewarding. Physical exhaustion told me I needed to say no and choose rest.
Moral distress signaled that I needed to fight for systemic change in
the ailing world around me.

In the past, I ignored these essential signals screaming at me until
they needed to ramp up their message with distressing mental and
physical health symptoms. I was only able to return to health when I
started paying attention to their vital information so I could manually
steer myself in new directions.

UNTRAINING OUR NEGATIVITY BIAS

While it's helpful to pay attention to the unpleasant experiences of our lives so we can approach them more skillfully, we don't need to dwell in the darkness all the time. We can also learn to rest in the awareness of our pleasant and neutral experiences.

Most of us don't tend to spend much time noticing these moments of respite. Instead, we get stuck focused on potential problems to ensure we don't miss any danger—what cognitive scientists call our *negativity bias*. It all goes back to our brain's life-saving function of focusing on survival rather than happiness. We've evolved to pay attention to every single potential threat in our lives while ignoring everything we perceive as safe.

Even if our mind can't find a problem in the present, it searches through the "if onlys" of the past or the "what ifs" of the future to find threats. Neuroscientists identified a specific network of our brain, the *default mode network*, that functions in this very task. It gets activated whenever we're not intentionally paying attention to our present-moment experience. When our mind rests or wanders—usually because it assesses the present moment as safe and not worthy of our attention—it quickly starts hunting for problems in the past and future. This default mode is also known as the *me-network*, because it's self-focused in nature, especially centering on personal failings and threats.

Like all the functions of our brains and bodies, there's nothing inherently bad about our default mode network. It helps us think about ourselves, others, and the world around us, providing perspective. But when we spend too much time in it—an imbalanced pattern we find when studying the brains of people experiencing episodes of depression and anxiety—we get stuck in our heads, leaving us less capable of acting in ways that solve our problems.[5]

I remember hiking alone in the desert one day. I interrupted the serenity of the present moment by looking far ahead toward the summit. I suddenly felt fear: from my vantage point, the trail ahead looked steep and dangerous. Then I looked behind me and panicked even more, as the trail below looked equally daunting. But when I looked down at the actual ground where I stood, I noticed the sturdiness of the footing all around me. I realized that each single step was safe. It's become my new motto when I'm anxious: This step is safe. We can overwhelm ourselves by thinking about all the threats in the future and past. But even in hard moments, our journey can feel more manageable when we focus on each single step in the present.

Learning to pay attention to our present-moment experiences can move our brain away from this default mode of problem-hunting through time and place, which leaves us chronically triggered into the inflammatory reactions of our stress response. We can find respite in the present—this one step—because it's always available to us, right here and now. While we can't control what experiences arise in our inner and outer worlds, we can control where we put our attention.

Thich Nhat Hanh taught a practice called "Touching the Earth," inviting us to feel the ground whenever we notice ourselves getting stuck in the default mode network. In this way, we can bring our full attention to anything in our present environment, opening our eyes to the living reality in front of us rather than getting lost in the dark alleys of the world of concepts.

"When walking past the cypress tree in the courtyard, we really see it. If we do not see the cypress in our own garden, how can we expect to see into our own true nature?" Hanh taught.[6] "This is why the master feels compassion every time her disciple asks a question about some Buddhist principles . . . 'This young man,' she thinks, 'still wishes to engage in the search for reality through concepts.' She does her best to extricate the student from the world of ideas and put him in the world of living reality. Look at the cypress in the courtyard! *Look at the cypress in the courtyard!*"

It's easier to keep our eyes open to the problems of the world and choose helpful actions if we don't get stuck permanently spinning out in them. We need to be both open to our distress signals and also flexible, so we can change the channel to more regulating experiences when we need respite to prevent overwhelming ourselves into panic or shutdown.

When we notice ourselves getting stuck in the dark alleys of thinking brains, a helpful way to move ourselves out of the default mode network is to shift our attention to whatever we are doing in the moment, what we call *mindfulness of daily living*. When we are eating, we can notice all the sensations—how it looks, smells, sounds, tastes, and feels—while we are eating. When we are showering, we can notice all the sensations of showering. Even when we are noticing ourselves thinking, we can notice the *process* of thinking and identify the thoughts, feelings, body sensations, and urges that arise, rather than getting lost in the content of the thoughts—time-traveling on a train of thought to the past and future.

When we're noticing ourselves spiraling in our heads or getting dysregulated, we can also move our attention to the external world, which can be more neutral when we're activated than noticing our inner experiences. A common exercise is 5–4–3–2–1. Here's one form of practicing this exercise:

Notice five sights we can see.
Notice four sensations we can feel.
Notice three sounds we can hear.
Notice two scents we can smell.
Notice one flavor we can taste.

This exercise can be modified in a variety of ways. It doesn't matter what numbers or senses you use. What is key is that you're getting out of your head and moving your awareness to what you sense in the present.

Another approach for getting out of our time-traveling heads is to move into our bodies (which we will explore in more detail in Chapter Six). While our mind loves to cling to the problems it perceives in the past and future, our body sensations live in the present. For example, when caught up in a stressful thought spiral, we can focus on the soles of our feet as we walk, because this part of our body is often quite neutral.

While the "self-care" industry encourages us to consume expensive products and services, we don't need to spend money to take respite in the present, nor do we even need to have a pleasurable activity to focus on. All we need is to be mindful of whatever is arising in our awareness right now.

When I facilitate mindfulness-based cognitive therapy groups, I invite participants to write down all the activities they do in a day and then, next to each activity, write down whether the activity is nourishing or depleting. We find that two things influence how nourishing an activity feels: our level of attention to the present moment and our attitude toward the activity.

In 2010, Harvard psychologists Matthew Killingsworth and Daniel Gilbert had participants track their happiness multiple times a day on smartphone apps. Not only did they find that participants spent over half their time in their default mode network—that is, thinking of something other than what was happening to them in the present—they also reported being much less happy when their minds were focused on the past or future.

What surprised the researchers most is that the participants' happiness had nothing to do with the activity they were engaged in, whether making love or working, but simply how much they were paying attention to what they were doing. The researchers discovered that paying attention in itself—regardless of whether an activity appears nourishing or depleting on the surface—may be the secret to happiness.

The attitude we bring to the activity also impacts how it's experienced. When we judge something as undesirable as we do it, we find it depleting, just like when we assume a medication will work, the placebo effect makes it work better. Similarly, the research on psychotherapy shows that a main indicator of how effective a therapy will be is our attitude toward it (and the relationship with our therapist). This research supports civil rights activist Maya Angelou's famous advice: If you don't like something, change it. If you can't change it, change your attitude.

Before my co-parent and I had kids, washing the dishes felt like a drag we wished to avoid. But during the hard early years of caring for our children, our attitudes shifted. We instead viewed doing the dishes as an opportunity to rest from the complex problems of the world and the big emotions of our screaming children, who depended on us to hold all that raw distress. Not only did we get the boost of feeling a sense of agency over one manageable task, but we used the moment to practice being in the present, observing the sensations of the warm water against our hands and the pressure of the dishes between our fingers. We didn't need to spend our paychecks on self-care luxuries that we couldn't afford. We simply had to change our attitude and awareness of what was right there in front of us. We only needed to look at the cypress tree.

I often read the poem "Do Not Ask Your Children to Strive" by William Martin to conclude this exercise in my groups. We do not need to ask our children to strive for extraordinary lives, Martin says. Instead, we can help them find the wonder and marvel in an ordinary life, "the joy of tasting tomatoes, apples and pears," the "infinite pleasure in the touch of a hand." When we make the ordinary come alive, he says, the extraordinary takes care of itself.

HOW STRIVING FOR HAPPINESS MAKES US MISERABLE

Too much joy, I swear, is lost in our desperation to keep it.
—OCEAN VUONG

"What if your very efforts to find happiness were actually preventing you from achieving it?" asks acceptance and commitment therapist Russ Harris in *The Happiness Trap*. The research agrees: the more we try to be happy, the less happy we actually are.

In 2011, a team of researchers led by Iris Mauss, director of the Emotion & Emotion Regulation Laboratory at the University of California, Berkeley, published two studies supporting this happiness paradox.[7] The first showed that participants who valued happiness the most reported half as many positive emotions and three-quarters more depressive symptoms than people who valued other things. They were also less satisfied with their lives. This echoes the research we explored in Chapter Three, where those who pursued hedonistic pleasures became more inflamed, while those focused on contributing to others became less inflamed.

In their second study, half of the participants were experimentally induced to value happiness by reading a false article on the science of happiness and then shown a funny movie clip. Those induced to value happiness enjoyed the clip the least.

Just down the coast, psychology professor Jonathan Schooler and his colleagues at the University of California, Santa Barbara, similarly found that when researchers instructed participants to "try to make yourself feel as happy as possible" while listening to a piece of music, they reported the opposite: they were less happy.[8]

Cognitive psychologists isolated a problem-solving function of our brain called *discrepancy-based processing*. Our minds compare the current state A to the desired state B, and then generate solutions for getting from A to B. While this approach works well for concrete challenges like changing a light bulb, it falls short when the problem is the gap between our painful emotional state and the happiness we assume we should feel.

Cognitive psychologists John Teasdale, Mark Williams, and Zindel Segal came together to integrate cognitive theory with mindfulness by creating the mindfulness-based cognitive therapy (MBCT) program. In their training manual, *Mindfulness-Based Cognitive Therapy for Depression*, they wrote:

To cope with waking in the morning feeling bad is difficult enough, but if we then match it against some standard, better mood, we worsen the very mood we wanted to get rid of. Soon, we find that the results of this "matching" process leads to a new train of thought: "I wish I didn't feel this bad. Why am I feeling this way? Why do I always feel this way?" . . . Our natural drive for happiness creates brooding and rumination: patterns of thinking, feeling and behaving that are unhelpful because they simply circle round and round, without producing a resolution, and making us feel worse.

Buddhist psychology diagnoses the source of our suffering as not the quality of our experiences themselves, but how we relate to them, especially by comparing each experience to an unrealistic standard of how we think it should be. In his first Noble Truth, the Buddha described *dukkha*, the inherent unsatisfactoriness, stress, or suffering in life—what cognitive scientists would call the current undesirable state A. In his second Noble Truth, the Buddha diagnosed the problem as habitually reacting to our experience with the natural desire for things to be different than how they actually are, thinking, *I should be happy* or *I shouldn't feel this way*, comparing state A to the desired state B. We move through the world with our minds giving automatic readouts of pleasant, unpleasant, or neutral.

If the experience is pleasant, we desperately cling to it, always anxious that it will end. If it's unpleasant, we try to push the experience away, hoping to rid ourselves of it. If it's neutral, we tune it out, missing out on the life that's right in front of us. As psychologist and mindfulness teacher Tara Brach says, "This leads to a perpetual treadmill race to nowhere, endlessly pounding after pleasure, endlessly fleeing from pain, and endlessly ignoring ninety percent of our experience."

The Buddha furthered this concept with his idea of the second arrow. The first arrow is shot at us—the difficult life or world event, the uncomfortable emotion or intrusive thought, the inherent pain or unsatisfactoriness of life. This we can't control. But then we shoot second arrows at ourselves with our own reactions to the pain, amplifying and prolonging it.

When we identify our experience as unpleasant, we can shoot second arrows with reactions of aversion and needing to get rid of it, feeling anxious that we are anxious, or angry when we feel shame; or judging ourselves for having a "bad" thought or urge, or ruminating about *Why me?*

I hesitate to mention the phrase "let it go," because it's so often misused to invalidate or push away our helpful emotional signals like anger, fear, and grief. We aren't trying to rid ourselves of emotions. But we do want to let go of the expectation that we should feel differently than what's already here.

When we identify our experience as pleasant, we can add second arrows with our anxious attachment to the experience. When watching our children or partner sleep at night, rather than experiencing the immense gratitude we feel toward them, we may get stuck in worries about all the potential ways we could lose them. Or we're so concerned that our weekend or time with a loved one is almost over that we stop enjoying the pleasant moment before us. To put it simply: pain is inevitable, but the second arrow of added suffering is optional.

In my mindfulness teacher training with Tara Brach, she told a story of a man whose therapist recommended he go to a retreat to feel better. At the retreat, as he departed from all the distractions of the modern world that constantly pulled him out of the present moment, he began to feel all the emotions that he'd been pushing away for years.

"I thought you said I was going to feel better at the retreat," he complained to his therapist when he returned. "You are feeling better," she responded. "You're feeling anger better and sadness better and fear better."

Practicing kind attention is not about blissing out or escaping to another world. It's not even a relaxation practice. Instead, we learn skills to better participate in the challenges that our current world presents to us, which require us to feel all the distressing signals so we can gather information about the challenges and our progress in order to solve them.

Bhante Henepola Gunaratana, a Sri Lankan Theravada Buddhist monk, teaches that mindfulness is learning not to cave in to the constant impulses of attachment and avoidance that urge us to choose immediate comfort. "The irony of it is that real peace comes only when you stop chasing it," he explains in *Mindfulness in Plain English*. He describes mindfulness as the mental art of stepping out of your own way, of facing reality fully to experience and accept life just as it is, while coping effectively with exactly what you find. While his students come to him expecting "instantaneous cosmic revelation, complete with angelic choirs," he says, "what they usually get is a more efficient way to take out the trash and better ways to deal with Uncle Herman."

ACCEPTANCE IS ACTIVE

It's not just bringing attention to our experiences that helps us cope in this challenging world; it's how we relate to them. "The dark thought, the shame, the malice, meet them at the door laughing, and invite them in," offered the Sufi mystic Rumi in his poem "The Guest House."

Tara Brach told us about a new problem that arose when the British colonists tried to play golf in Kolkata: the monkeys would steal the balls as they played. The golfers tried everything to rid themselves of the problem. They built high fences around the course, but the monkeys climbed over them. They hired vans to transport the monkeys away, but the monkeys kept coming back. Finally, exasperated, they decided on a new rule: play the ball wherever the monkey drops it.

As Brach taught, rather than fighting the "endless and fruitless battle for control," can we play the ball of life wherever it lands? Whether it's a layoff at work, an illness, or a divorce, we must accept the reality of the present moment—letting go of the expectation that it should be different—to respond skillfully to what's already here.

Here's an exercise to try out this stance yourself:

1. FIRST, let's practice noticing all of our inner experiences—the thoughts, feelings, body sensations, and urges to act—that arise within our awareness. Each time we become aware of an experience within us, we can see what happens when we say no to it, noticing what arises next with this reaction.

   ▪ We usually notice how the intensity of these unwanted experiences increases when we try to push them away with a no.

2. THEN, we can try the opposite approach, saying yes to these experiences whenever they arise. "Not *Yes, I like it* or *Yes, stay forever*, but, *Yes, it's already here, let me be with it*," Brach taught me. It's about acknowledging and allowing whatever's arising in each moment, without trying to make it different than what it is.

   ▪ When we practice meeting our inner experiences with a yes, we usually notice that they become less distressing, passing through us faster and with more ease.

Many people presume that acceptance is a passive submission, a surrender without a fight to the harms in our outer worlds. I'm not suggesting that we accept all the injustices and preventable disorders in our outer world without trying to change them. But acceptance is a vital first step to action. We need to accept what's already here, and all the alarms arising within our bodies in response to the outer problems— our uncomfortable emotions, body sensations, thoughts, and urges to act—before we can see the problem clearly enough to change it.

If the colonizers had paid more attention to the countless frustration alarms arising when they tried to play golf in Kolkata, they could have seen the bigger picture more clearly: occupying and creating a golf course on land they weren't educated on and where they weren't welcome wasn't a good idea. So, the first step is to accept that the monkeys are moving the balls, but the second step is to look even

deeper to explore what important lesson this discomfort may be signaling. Sometimes, it's just bad luck; at other times, it's signaling that
we're on the wrong path and need to pivot.

A key question to ask ourselves is whether a problem in our external
world is within our control to solve. At times, we are empowered enough
to change the situation, but we're missing the opportunity because we
aren't accepting or able to hold the inner feelings, such as our immense
guilt or grief and their painful body sensations. When we build skills
to embrace and tolerate these inner experiences, we find we're able to
hold the reality of our outer worlds long enough to improve them, even
if it's one small step at a time. In the next chapters, we'll explore skills to
more comfortably hold all of these inner experiences.

COMPASSION IS A PRACTICE

Don't meditate to fix yourself, to heal yourself, to improve
yourself, to redeem yourself; rather, do it as an act of love, of
deep warm friendship to yourself. In this way there is no longer
any need for the subtle aggression of self-improvement, for the
endless guilt of not doing enough. It offers the possibility of
an end to the ceaseless round of trying so hard that wraps so
many people's lives in a knot. Instead, there is now meditation
as an act of love. How endlessly delightful and encouraging.

—Bob Sharples

When I spent a week learning self-compassion practices in the
deserts of California from the founders of Mindful Self-Compassion
(MSC), Kristin Neff, a professor and researcher at the University of
Texas, and Christopher Germer, a psychologist at Harvard, they introduced a simple exercise that I've since shared with countless people.

First, they had us think about a time in our lives when a close
friend or loved one experienced some sort of failure or hardship and
imagine how we would respond to them. What type of things would

we say and with what tone would we communicate it? Go ahead and try this for yourself.

Oh love, this is so hard. I'm here with you. It makes so much sense you hurt. You are so much more than this one thing. This doesn't change how much I love and cherish you. So much of this was out of your control. It will get better. Should we get ice cream or dance it out?

Then, we imagined that the same failure or hardship happened to ourselves. What would we say to ourselves? And what tone would we use?

I'm such a screwup. I always mess things up. How could I have been so stupid? This is all my fault. I'm always going to be a failure. I can't let others know how bad I am.

I've facilitated this exercise for over a decade, and all my participants report the same conclusion: we usually have critical thoughts toward ourselves, but kind and generous ones toward those we love. The moment I ask participants to write down what they would say to themselves, the room breaks out in laughter, because it's so painfully obvious how differently we treat our friends and ourselves in the exact same situation.

The great news is that we don't need to learn the skill of compassion from scratch. We just need to give ourselves permission to direct this kindness toward ourselves. Just as we likely have no reservations about bandaging a cut when we're bleeding, we can learn to treat our emotional wounds with the same tenderness. Part of learning self-compassion is internalizing the voice of this caring, kind friend who accepts and makes sense of the pain without judgment. Neff describes self-compassion as paying attention to our own suffering, recognizing it as part of the human condition, and then offering kindness to these hurting places. It's about creating a healthy relationship with our own experiences of pain and vulnerability. Compassion is often described as *when love meets pain*.

Giving ourselves permission to practice self-compassion isn't easy. "When I talked with friends and acquaintances about self-love, I was surprised to see how many of us feel troubled by the notion, as though the very idea implies too much narcissism or selfishness," wrote bell hooks, a social activist and professor at Berea College who studied race, feminism, and class.[9] "We need to stop fearfully equating it with self-centeredness and selfishness. Self-love is the foundation of our loving practice . . . When we give this precious gift to ourselves, we are able to reach out to others from a place of fullness and not from a place of lack." We often believe that we only have a finite amount of love or compassion to offer, so we should save it all for other people. But compassion and love are contagious. The more we offer it to ourselves or others, the more we have to offer again.

"But I need to be harder on myself because I'm responsible for my own growth and improvement," many of my group participants argue. Would you pay a therapist to say those critical things to you in the name of self-improvement? Would you really find that response helpful?

I can answer that with the research: criticizing ourselves or others won't improve performance, or anything for that matter. Instead, reviews of the research link self-compassion to less stress, anxiety, and depression,[10] better resilience in the face of negative life events,[11] and more feelings of happiness, optimism, gratitude, autonomy, competence, connectedness to others, self-determination, emotional intelligence, wisdom, initiative, curiosity, flexibility, and life satisfaction.[12] As a psychiatrist who's studied many treatment options, I find nothing more impressive than the research outcomes for compassion.

THE HOLLOW PROMISE OF SELF-ESTEEM

For years, boosting self-esteem dominated the Western mental health scene as a popular pursuit on the path to wellness. Intuitively, we believed that high self-esteem—defined as our perception of our own value—would improve our lives. But when I attended Kristin Neff's training on self-compassion, she explained that self-compassion and self-esteem are different concepts.

Neff taught us that many studies do link high self-esteem to happiness, improved initiative, and persistence after failing.[13] And low self-esteem can relate to depression, low motivation, and suicidal thoughts.[14] Yet despite widespread enthusiasm for improving self-esteem in schools, workplaces, and mental health clinics alike, interventions hoping to improve our self-esteem haven't panned out.[15]

First, studies show that self-esteem is highly resistant to change, so it's very hard to boost it. Second, high self-esteem doesn't improve relationships or work and school performance; rather, it's simply the result of good performance. And while people with high self-esteem may perceive themselves to be more likable and have better relationships, there is no link between self-esteem and the quality or duration of their relationships. In fact, high self-esteem can lead to entitlement, self-absorption, and a lack of concern for others, which repels others.

The problem with self-esteem, Neff taught, is that it involves splitting the collective by comparing ourselves to others.[16] The need to boost self-esteem may cause us to compete with and see the worst in each other so that we can compare ourselves more favorably, leading to behaviors of dominance, division, and dehumanization.[17]

Having a healthy relationship with ourselves, however, is still essential to our wellness. That's where the concept of self-compassion comes in. Rather than needing to compare and separate ourselves from the pack to establish our self-worth, we take solace in our shared struggles as part of the common human condition. In this way, we can offer gentle kindness to these hurting parts that live in us all.

Failures, flaws, and pain are inevitable for everyone at different times in our lives. But our pain doesn't need to be personal. While we all have different histories and flavors of pain, we all suffer, and we're all ruled by unconscious forces that cause us to make many mistakes. So, instead of the fiction of comparing ourselves as better than everyone else to maintain our self-esteem, we can take comfort in knowing that we share in the human condition of regularly experiencing suffering, pain, and imperfections, just like everyone else.

Self-compassion doesn't imply passivity or resignation. It can be the most active path to helpful action. Rather than blaming or shaming ourselves to change, which pushes us toward denial, avoidance, and shutting down, acceptance and nonjudgment toward our messy parts frees us to pay attention to what needs to change. And self-compassion creates a soft landing when we inevitably need it. It also moves us from our threat network to our care system, allowing us to regain access to the higher parts of our brain in the prefrontal cortex so we can make more helpful, reflective actions in line with our values.

Luckily, we can improve self-compassion with practice. Neff's research shows that even a few weeks of self-compassion practice decreases suffering and improves wellness. With neuroplasticity, we can create new, healthier paths in our brain. Neuroscientists say, "What fires together wires together," meaning that habits of thinking, feeling, and acting become repetitive and easy patterns to follow again, reflected by the wirings of the neurons in our brains. Our brains are like a forest with many paths, and we often tend to reactively take the most well-trodden trails, because that's the path of least resistance.

When we try to create a new, healthier path, it can often feel like bushwhacking at the beginning—an awkward slog through the thick undergrowth of sticks and plants and mud. But over time, as we try this new path again and again, we smooth out a healthier path of least resistance—our autopilot—as our neurons begin to wire this way. As Brené Brown points out, compassion isn't something you have or don't have; it's a commitment you choose to practice.[18] And with practice, we can rewire our brains so that compassion becomes our new autopilot.

Self-compassion is a portable source of support, available twenty-four hours a day, seven days a week—even when all of our friends and family are unavailable. Neff offers many exercises to help us develop the habit of self-compassion in her books *Self-Compassion, Fierce Self-Compassion*, and *The Mindful Self-Compassion Workbook*, the latter coauthored with Chris Germer. Neff's self-compassion break includes three steps to practicing self-compassion. You can also practice these steps when offering others compassion.

SELF-COMPASSION BREAK[19]

1. **BRING AWARENESS TO SUFFERING.** For example, you may say to yourself, *This is a moment of suffering; This hurts; This is tough.* As best you can, gently observe and label inner experiences such as thoughts, feelings, body sensations, or urges to act, allowing them to be there without judgment.

2. **RECOGNIZE THAT THESE INNER EXPERIENCES ARE PART OF THE COMMON HUMAN CONDITION, AND THAT SUFFERING IS A NORMAL PART OF LIFE.** For example, *This is being human; Other people feel this way, I'm not alone; We all struggle in our lives.*

3. **EXTEND KINDNESS OR TENDERNESS.** *Experiment with what expression of kindness is the best fit for you, whether it's offering kind words to yourself, gentle touch, the gift of a moment to yourself or a cup of tea, or offering yourself a hot bath or time to be mindful in nature.*

Practicing self-compassion doesn't always feel warm and fuzzy. Sometimes, the act of offering ourselves kindness brings up an eruption of tears, shame, or sadness, the opposite of what we'd expect to experience. Neff identifies this reaction as *back draft*, a term used in firefighting to describe how we can ignite a fire further by offering a gush of oxygen from opening a window or door. When we experience kindness, we may be reminded of all the times we didn't receive kindness in our past, fueling the pain further and intensifying it.

If this happens, we can shift to practicing self-compassion in gradual, smaller doses and acknowledge the back draft as it arises, without needing it to be any different than it is. If it feels overwhelming, we can pivot to practicing some of the grounding exercises, such as soles of the feet, 5–4–3–2–1, those offered in the next chapters, or find the support of a mental health professional or loved one.

A HEALTHY DOSE OF COMPASSION

"If you want others to be happy, practice compassion," teaches the Dalai Lama. "If you want to be happy, practice compassion." Yet in helping professions, we often speak of the burnout of *compassion fatigue,* when we take in too much suffering from others. But compassion fatigue is a misnomer: researchers have shown that compassion doesn't fatigue.[20] But empathy can.

Neurophysiologist Giacomo Rizzolatti stumbled upon mirror neurons accidentally while studying the brain functions of monkeys. As he reached for something, he noticed a burst of neural activity in the monkeys' brains that mimicked his own actions, even though the monkeys weren't moving themselves. He discovered that these neurons mirror the neural firings of others, helping us to feel, understand, and imitate the inner experiences of those around us.[21]

When our wonderful mirror neurons allow us to feel what others are feeling, we can also experience *empathic distress*, pushing us into the same fight, flight, or freeze states if we don't have the skills to cope with the emotions. If we're feeling such empathic distress every day, we can deplete our inner resources, leading to *empathy fatigue* or burnout. But empathy doesn't have to be distressing, just like experiencing all our healthy emotions doesn't have to cause suffering.

Empathy can also lead to *empathic concern* when we use the strategies we're learning now to hold the distressing emotions with kind attention and compassion, without evaluating them as bad, personal, or permanent. If we practice compassion when feeling others' distress, we end up experiencing pleasant feelings, connection, and better health. Just like we're learning to skillfully hold our own passing emotions, thoughts, urges, and body sensations with kind attention, we can also practice these same skills when feeling someone else's emotions, so we don't personalize these feelings and experience them as our own.[22]

For example, when so many of us face evidence of children being harmed by war or family violence, we may fuse with the immense feelings of their distress, pushing us into a flight or freeze response. We might notice that we're unable to read certain news stories or watch clips of what's happening around the world. Instead, we may turn away to protect ourselves from these scary feelings and fail to acknowledge the danger or help them. This is *empathic distress*, when we can't separate our self from the emotions of others, causing an increased sense of threat, pain, and activation on brain scans.[23]

But if we don't blur the self-other boundary, we can still notice and feel the distressing emotions arising within our bodies and use this important emotional signal to motivate us to offer compassion and help them. While empathy is feeling with someone, compassion is feeling for them, with care and concern.[24] Just like self-compassion describes *how* we relate tenderly to our own distress, compassion describes how we relate tenderly to the distress we empathically feel from others. We move ourselves out of the threat systems that the other person is feeling and instead engage our care networks, pumping out the caregiving and bonding hormone, oxytocin.

As we discussed in Chapter Three, this *tend-and-befriend* care system can overpower our *fight-or-flight* threat signaling. Studies show that when we extend compassion to others in pain, our neural networks associated with rewards, positive emotions, and bonding light up, making us feel better.[25] Just like with self-compassion training, the more we practice compassion toward others, the more we wire our neural pathways in this healthy direction and the easier it becomes to help and support others.[26]

CULTIVATING COLLECTIVE COMPASSION

Compassion is the keen awareness of the
interdependence of all things.
—THOMAS MERTON

Thich Nhat Hanh started the engaged Buddhism movement in Vietnam, advocating for this kind attention, acceptance, and compassion to be present everywhere, not just in the temple. "It is with that kind of peace and stability that you can serve," he explained. "It's not about 'doing' something; it's about 'being' something—being peace, being hope, being solid. Every action will come out of that, because peace, stability, and freedom always seek a way to express themselves in action."

As our world becomes increasingly dysregulated and divided, it's getting harder to access compassion. "In the first step towards a compassionate heart, we must develop our empathy and closeness to others," teaches the Dalai Lama.[27] "We must recognize the gravity of their misery. The closer we are to a person, the more unbearable we find that person's suffering."

Yet our individualist cultures and internalized dynamics of domination, division, and indifference make us feel distant from the people our actions are impacting. It becomes even more challenging when stress deactivates our prefrontal cortex, so we no longer have access to its functions of empathy and compassion. We lose our capacity to see that our denial of climate change is killing others across the world through fires, droughts, and storms. Nor can we see that the inequities we benefit from are starving others and making us all sick.

The Dalai Lama invites us to reflect on our food, clothes, homes, city's infrastructure, and all the other resources and needs that others provide for us to recognize our interconnection.[28] For example, with each bite of bread, we can imagine where the seeds come from, who planted, watered, weeded, harvested, processed, transported, packaged, stored, and sold the grains that were then combined with other ingredients that each came from other people's labor and investments, by someone who baked, processed, transported, and so on. We can similarly think of the processes involved in the clothes we wear and the buildings we visit. Or all the people who researched, studied, and taught generations of healers to offer us a ceremony, flu shot, acupuncture session, massage, or medicine. It would be impossible to count all the people involved in each and every thing we need to survive.

"A flower is full of everything in the cosmos—sunshine, clouds, air, and space," Thich Nhat Hanh explained.[29] "It is empty of only one thing: a separate self. But when you have touched the nature of interbeing of the flower, you truly see the flower. If you see a person and don't also see his society, education, ancestors, culture, and environment, you have not really seen that person."

Because our ancestors and future generations are always present within us, liberation is not an individual matter, Hahn explained. When we take a mindful step, for example, we can visualize others, near and far, in the past or future, walking along with us. We can offer compassion to our ancestors, understanding that they may not have had the chance to learn the practices of kind awareness and compassion that have helped us, and we can also offer compassion to future generations who may face similar pains and challenges.

Rather than judging others for not having these skills, we can offer them an extra dose of compassion for their lack of access to such teachings or the safety to be regulated enough to practice them. "As you begin to walk for dear ones, you can walk for the people who have made your life miserable. You can walk for those who have attacked you, who have destroyed your home, your country, and your people," taught Hahn. "These people weren't happy. They didn't have enough love for themselves and for other people . . . If your step can bring you more stability and freedom, then you are serving the world. It is with that kind of peace and stability that you can serve."

At the 2024 Vancouver Writer's Fest, when Jewish-Canadian Gabor Maté joined Palestinian-Canadian Raja G. Khouri to discuss the grief and trauma in Israel and Palestine, Maté explained that the conflict is not about Jews or Palestinians but about who has lost touch with humanity and who has not. The most common casualty of the war is that we've lost the capacity to grieve for the other, said Khouri. The moderator, CBC Radio host Elamin Abdelmahmoud, added that we've been pushed to pick a side to feel compassion for, that even grieving feels political, and in doing so, we're severing ourselves from our own humanity. When we can't see the sacred humanity in others—and stand up for everyone's rights to safety, dignity, and justice—we lose our own.

What struck me most about this almost two-hour live conversation was how Maté, Khouri, Abdelmahmoud, the audience members asking questions, and the hundreds of people witnessing the discussion stayed entirely regulated and compassionate with every comment, despite it being about one of the most polarizing atrocities facing our collective right now.

When we offer kind attention to our present-moment experiences, we can allow the grief and anger to arise in awareness and channel its energy to fuel the action needed to bring the world back into balance. We can stop clinging to identities that rob us of our compassion for others and instead heal our humanity by standing up against the injustices that harm us all.

PUTTING IT ALL INTO PRACTICE

There are many different ways to practice kind attention. We can start by focusing on a single anchor to the present moment, such as noticing each breath or step. Then, we can build our brain's flexibility and balance by shifting our attention between different anchors to the present moment, including any of the following senses:

Note: When we're activated, it can often be more comfortable to begin with observing the external senses, because it's easier to perceive them as not personal.

1. SENSING the Outer World:

   SOUND: Noticing the pitch, tone, volume of different sounds arising and passing within your awareness (rather than thinking about the sounds).

   SIGHT: Noticing the colors, shapes, and textures of objects around you.

   SMELL: Noticing the different scents or odors.

   TASTE: Noticing the complex flavors.

   TOUCH: Noticing the sensations of the external world touching your body.

2. BODY Sensations:

   BREATH: Observing the dance of body sensations as the breath moves in and out of the body. You can try zooming into the sensations of areas where the breath is most vivid to you, or zooming out to notice the body as a whole breathing.

   MINDFULNESS OF BODY SENSATIONS AT REST: Zooming out to feel the body as a whole, or zooming in, as if we have a spotlight investigating the felt sensations of specific parts of the body. This can also be done systematically, like a body scan, moving from head to toe.

   MINDFULNESS OF MOVEMENT: In the same way, noticing the internal sensations of our body in motion.

3. THOUGHTS: Noticing the thoughts arising and passing, identifying thoughts as thoughts, trying not to get caught up in their content or push them away.

4. FEELINGS: Noticing what emotional signals are present and how they are expressed in the body.

5. INTERCONNECTEDNESS: Observing our sense of connection to others and our environment, perhaps offering loving kindness or compassion in whatever way feels authentic.

CREATING BALANCE IN ALL OUR SYSTEMS

These kinds of exercises help integrate our nervous systems so that no one part—the mind, body, internal, external, self, or others—dominates or splits off from our attention. Just like the larger systems in our outer worlds, we need our nervous systems to be flexible, communicating, and in balance.

But sometimes, kind attention isn't enough to keep us regulated, especially when the world feels like a dumpster fire. In the next chapter, we'll dive into more strategies to help us regulate our emotions in the chaos—at least most of the time. In certain situations we need to accept that sometimes we're all a hot mess. And some situations require all our alarms to scream so we finally pay attention to the problem long enough to fix it.

SIX

DE-HIJACKING OUR BRAINS

> People will forget what you said, people will forget what you
> did, but people will never forget how you made them feel.
> —MAYA ANGELOU

_____

MANY OF US ARE CONFUSED AS TO WHY OUR COLLECTIVES KEEP ACTING IN WAYS THAT spiral us toward escalating disorder, especially when we know what our systems need to return to balance.

While we've explored how our nervous systems are marvelously adapted to our environments to meet our needs, keep us safe, and return our systems to balance, there's a glaring weak spot in their design: they can be hijacked.

Freedom House's _2024 Freedom in the World_ report found that 40 percent of the global population experienced a decline in freedom, dropping for the nineteenth year in a row, with political rights and civil liberties diminished in fifty-two countries. One of the biggest threats facing democracies around the world, they identified, is elected leaders undermining democratic institutions, such as the justice system, free press, and many other regulating structures that keep our systems in balance.

Even in countries where we have the apparent freedom and safety to vote, many election results leave us puzzled as to why so many of us appear to vote against our own best interests. While it's tempting to denounce one another if we don't agree with each other's politics, no one is stupid or bad, even when we're acting in unhealthy ways. We all just have times when our higher brain's prefrontal cortex—the part that functions in complex reasoning, such as considering long-term consequences, values, and other perspectives—is deactivated by stress.

It's not that any of us are willfully choosing to act and think in unhelpful ways; it's just that in these moments of dysregulation, we simply don't have the capacity to access our higher brain functions to consider the needs of our future health.

In *The Shock Doctrine,* Naomi Klein offers countless examples of political actors exploiting or creating crises to hijack our brains with stress. Then they can push through undesirable policies that further imbalance our systems by favoring the interests of the political and corporate elite, while disadvantaging and disenfranchising everyone else. In this way, they maintain the cancerous dynamics of dominance, division, and indifference in our social systems.

The rise of social media has detonated our dysregulation even more with the constant shocks of divisive misinformation and lies. We don't need to steal an election by hacking a voting booth. We can simply hijack the voters' brains so they lose their capacity to think about diverse perspectives, consider long-term consequences, or access trust, creativity, and compassion.

In this frightened state, we don't trust in *we* anymore. It's every person for themselves. When we're regulated, there's nothing more unattractive than lying, bullying, and self-promoting behaviors. But when we're pushed into our stress response, the messages of distrusting others, focusing only on oneself, and being saved by an all-knowing supreme leader match our state of dysregulation.

Since we operate on a negativity bias to ensure we don't miss any trace of danger, it's a lot easier to dysregulate someone than to co-regulate them. And nothing is more contagious than dysregulation.

When my colleagues and I developed our Raising Resilient Kids program, we offered caregivers a variety of skills to manage the many rocky moments when our children (or co-parents) become emotionally dysregulated. It's so tempting to try to persuade others to get their prefrontal cortex back online with rational arguments, such as how unlikely it is that a feared event will actually occur, or to suggest that they consider someone else's feelings. Or we try to convince them to behave in more helpful ways by taking away their privileges or canceling a positive future event.

But these interventions don't work when we're emotionally dysregulated. Our prefrontal cortex shuts off, so we can't think logically, process long-term consequences, or consider the needs and perspectives of others. We first need to bring our higher brain functions back online. We need to feel safe and have our dysregulation recognized with compassion. And we need the co-regulation of someone who's regulated themselves. Only then can we learn to self-regulate with practices that will help us regain access to our capacity to think and act in ways that will support our long-term wellness.

When we understand how easy it is for all of our systems to dysregulate, we can learn to identify when we're activated or shut down, and then practice a variety of skills to both help ourselves and others come back online so we can defend ourselves against attacks to the health of our collective.

While our nations often focus on building the security of strong borders and economies, our safety depends more on the strength of our capacity for equanimity—the ability of us all to regulate, cooperate, and act in line with our values under the pressure of the world's escalating dysregulation.

SEEING WHAT'S HAPPENING

My training in mindfulness comes from the lineage of Vipassana Buddhism, known as *mindfulness* or *insight meditation*. Over 2,500 years ago, the Buddha invited others to experience the teachings of Vipassana as a path to self-discovery. He didn't tell people what to believe, but suggested they try cultivating a gentle awareness of their own experiences to investigate the true nature of reality for themselves.[1]

When we repeatedly pay attention to our own experiences, we can't help but notice certain insights arising. We discover the inherent unsatisfactoriness of everyday life. We realize how much effort we expend clinging to comfort while pushing away distress, instead of learning to listen to the urgent information emerging from our awareness, all while surfing the ever-passing waves of discomfort that it brings. As we keep observing, we see that life is uncomfortable, even when we're doing it right. Accepting the truth of life's inevitable pain can reduce the added suffering we layer on to it by assuming that it should be different.

A second insight we observe as we continue to pay close attention to reality is that every experience is impermanent, always changing before us. Not only is our external world constantly in flux—the people and systems we depend on get sick, die, move, or change—but we start to see that our intense feelings of being activated into fight-or-flight or deactivated into freeze are also fleeting. And we notice that each emotional state is accompanied by associated storylines and specific beliefs, powerful urges to react, and distressing body sensations that all completely change as they arise and then pass again, in a dynamic, ever-flowing dance.

When I first thought about impermanence, I became more anxious, seeing it as a threat that stole away my last withering sense of certainty in this scary world. I needed to hold on to something—a stable relationship, my sense of self, health, faith in justice or democracy, the survival of our species—to anchor me into some sense of certainty within this chaotic world.

But the reality that everything's impermanent wasn't the real source of my anxiety. My anxiety developed from desperately clinging to the delusion that things should stay the same. As I continued to practice kind attention, I realized that observing everything's impermanence soothed me in ways that the fantasy of clinging to any one certain thing never could. My anchor became awareness itself: even when the weather of life kept changing, my capacity to gently observe and have gratitude for each present-moment experience stayed the same.

The reality of impermanence relates to the final insight of no self, that even what we consider as static as our sense of self is always changing. Just as the cells that we're made of are constantly replaced with new ones, our thoughts, feelings, body sensations, and urges come and go in response to our environments, biology, and past learning. There is no static entity that we can call our self. As we begin to observe our habits closely and become more flexible and skillful in choosing different responses, even our stuck patterns of behaving, thinking, and feeling, which define our personalities, change as they become more responsive to the unique needs of new situations.

In this way, Dan Siegel taught me to say, "I lead with this pattern" of thinking, feeling, and behaving that we consider a personality trait to prevent us from getting stuck in a rigid identity. He describes these patterns of personality as a prison when we fuse with them, where past adversities and learning force us to act in fixed and limited ways. Jaak Panskepp's research similarly shows that our individual subcortical networks of seeking, care, lust, rage, fear, separation distress, and play can become rigidly sensitized or desensitized, pushing us to depend more on one system and less on another, as we adapt to environmental stress.

When we experience oppression or abuse, resources are not distributed equally, or when we live in systems of injustice, our rage circuitry often becomes sensitized, because we might need to engage our fight mode more often to survive this hostile environment. Or if we're exposed to constant uncertainty and threats to our safety, our fear pathways may become sensitized, pushing us to lead with flight mode's pattern of hypervigilance, catastrophic thinking, or avoidance. If our bonding needs haven't been met, our separation distress network might become either sensitized or desensitized, so we lead with a pattern of our fawning mode's attachment anxiety or flight or freeze mode's avoidance. Or if we're constantly facing a world of low rewards, our seeking, lust, and play pathways may become desensitized, leading with a freeze pattern of apathy or the need for substances or other addictive behaviors to cope.

Our journey to wellness allows us to loosen the rigid dominance of only one pattern of thinking, feeling, and acting, so we have a wider array of responses available to us to meet the unique needs of each new situation. "Personality can be thought of as something that keeps us from the reality of who we really are," Dan Siegel taught me. And who we really are is the one who observes all these ever-changing mental states, the grounded mountain that can witness and hold it all. No thought, feeling, urge, or body sensation defines us, even when we're stuck in stress or trauma cycles that keep us circling in the same alarm networks. All of us can have these experiences when we're faced with enough stress. And all of us can think, feel, and act markedly differently when our environments support justice, safety, and care.

Studies show that when we're younger or haven't had the opportunity to pay attention to how our inner experiences come and go over time, we're more prone to personalize our thoughts, feelings, and behaviors, attaching them more to a fixed sense of self.[2] As we age, we identify less with our internal experiences because we've spent years observing them fluctuate, and we realize that everything is constantly changing both inside and outside of ourselves. We can accelerate this learning by paying closer attention now, realizing that our thoughts, feelings, body sensations, and urges are impermanent inner experiences that constantly arise and pass. They don't define our worth or our identity. When we take everything less personally, we don't need to add so many second arrows of blame and shame when any of us flip into fawn, fight, flight, or freeze reactions.

While it's often hard not to fuse our identities with our passing experiences when pushed into a stress response, we can learn to offer gentleness to ourselves and others afterward, once we've had a

chance to regulate and come back online. We all find ourselves believing judgmental stories of ourselves and others when activated, but
when we regulate in safety and connection, these stories can then be
reprocessed with our prefrontal cortex's capacity for nonidentification,
empathy, and compassion. It's not the rupture that matters in the long
run, but how well we repair it. When we practice kind awareness and
hold all these changing experiences lightly, we become more capable
of being with the problems in our world so we can focus on them long
enough to fix them.

After much practice, my partner and I find it easy to bring up
difficult feelings and conflicts in real time, because we both trust that
we're on the same team and want the best for each other. When we
inevitably act in ways that upset the other, we talk about the thoughts,
feelings, and action urges that are passing through us with care, naming when we've slipped into fawn, fight, flight, or freeze—we know
that nothing's wrong with us for acting and reacting as we do. We
might notice when our reactions are false alarms, reflecting old stories
internalized from our pasts. Or we might be curious if our current
alarms are ringing to alert us to present problems that need addressing.

Even when we get triggered into our stress responses and act
in unhelpful ways, we need to remember that it's not personal, even
when it's messy. We're simply bumbling humans trying our best with
trigger-happy alarm systems wired into our bodies to survive. We
can recover by compassionately labeling that we've slipped into these
states and lost access to our higher brain's prefrontal cortex functions.
But we must remember that we can't rationalize with each other when
in this state. No amount of reasoning with facts, consequences, or
hopes of understanding another's perspective will talk us out of it—
these strategies can get us more rigidly stuck in our stress responses if
we feel more threatened in the process. When pushed offline, we can't
register the evidence of how inequities, injustices, and bullying, or the
collapse of our climate, deadly pandemics, and violent dehumaniza-

tion will harm us all. Instead, we first need to help each other feel safe enough to turn off our threat responses and come back online.

But so many of us don't have the option of choosing safety right now: our families, partners, schools, workplaces, communities, leaders, or global crises keep punting us down the steps of our defense system to live in a persistent state of dysregulation. When we're exposed to chronic and extreme stress, such as when facing ongoing conflict, oppression, or poverty, we can live in our fawn, fight, flight, or freeze responses for so long that it feels like our personality or culture. You can see how we might label people living in toxic relationships or environments as submissive and inauthentic (fawn), demanding and hostile (fight), anxious and avoidant (flight), or passive and cold (freeze). But these reactions are still fleeting, although repetitive, reactions to stress.

We can observe all these reactions within ourselves, others, and our collectives when faced with the right stressor. Our bodies and minds create all sorts of inner experiences in response to our environments. And once we start to take everything less personally, we have the power to accept all these things so we can change what's within our power to improve.

While it might be tempting to wish we could stay in balance all the time, we wouldn't be responding appropriately to our dynamic environments. We need all of our protective systems to keep us safe. We can learn to recognize what protective state we are in and move flexibly between states to match the needs of the situation, rather than make the situation worse by denying, judging, or trying to push these defenses away.

BEFRIENDING OUR SURVIVAL SYSTEM

"I've always known that I carry my past with me, but it exists in moods and flashes. A raised hand, a bitten tongue, a moment of terror," wrote journalist Stephanie Foo in her memoir *What My Bones Know*. For years, Foo suffered from the constant distress and dissociation of her reactive nervous system that kept her stuck in states of fight, flight, or freeze. Then one day, she listened to a podcast featuring psychologist Jacob Ham, the director of Mount Sinai's Center for Child Trauma and Resilience.

Ham likened our stress reactions to the Hulk. "As his rage grows, his IQ decreases. He can't speak, he can't form complete thoughts, he loses self-awareness," Foo says. "All he cares about is what's in front of him and how he can protect himself. And he can't turn the Hulk off immediately—it takes time for him to calm down, to sleep it off." But the Hulk is not a villain, Ham explained in Foo's headphones. "He's actually one of the most badass superheroes in the whole universe," he said.

Foo was all too familiar with our habit of judging our inner Hulk when it's activated, thinking to ourselves, *Oh no. I'm losing control and turning into a monster again. No, stop! Hulk, go away!* Yet the more we fight or fear these states, the further we push ourselves into them as our harsh interpretations of our reactions become a new threat to fear or fight, creating a vicious cycle.

Instead, Ham taught Foo the opposite approach: to talk to her own Hulk tenderly. Rather than see it as a threat that scares her even more, she can see her Hulk as a safety response that protects her. Ham encourages us to instead say, *Hulk, you're back? You think I'm in trouble? Oh, thank you so much for loving me so much that you're trying to protect me.* "To frame it in this way was comforting," Foo wrote, "that rage is not always evil." Instead, it can be productive if used correctly.

Foo immediately emailed Ham for an interview. They decided to record working together in therapy so she could better illustrate its process to the public. In therapy, Ham helped Foo tenderly observe and identify her own states of activation and shutdown. He'd point out the times when she became hypervigilant or dismissive, and also the times when it felt easy to resonate with her, as she seemed more alive and connected to her emotions. "I'm just trying to point out things for you to wonder about," Ham told her. "We're going to keep practicing curiosity and exploration rather than judgment, and it's through this process you'll start being nicer to yourself."

Foo made deep progress in this style of psychodynamic therapy, describing it as an interesting project to investigate rather than a depressing way to obsess over her flaws. Working with Ham made Foo's activated and shutdown states feel less personal. Just like working with her editors on journalism pieces, "We were collaborating to make my work better."

We can learn to offer ourselves this same kind attention to our inner states to build our capacity to be gentle with our badass inner superheroes. When we experience trauma or notice persistent states of dysregulation that are difficult to soothe on our own, we often need the co-regulation and support of someone else to help us learn these skills, which we will discuss in Chapter Nine. The help of a partner, peer, adviser, elder, or therapist can support us in learning to be kind with these experiences as we identify all our very normal stressed-out states, even when they're not pretty.

NOTICING WHERE WE ARE ON THE DIAL OF ACTIVATION

Comedian Trevor Noah grew up in South Africa during apartheid, when his very existence as a child of a Black mom and white father was illegal, requiring him and his single mother to live in a heightened state of hypervigilance and hiding to survive the oppressive regime. In his memoir, *Born a Crime*, Noah describes how his healthy adaptation of a sensitized flight response saved his life.

When he was nine years old, the driver of a minibus once made many racist comments toward his mom, calling her a "disgusting woman," because of her Xhosa identity. As the man escalated, adding, "Tonight you're going to learn your lesson," his mom suddenly threw Noah out of the car, yelling "Run!" as she jumped through the open door after him, cradling his baby brother in her arms. Noah wrote:

So I ran, and she ran, and nobody ran like me and my mom.
It's weird to explain, but I just knew what to do. It was animal
instinct, learned in a world where violence was always lurking
and waiting to erupt. In the townships, when the police came
swooping in with their riot gear and armored cars and helicopters,
I knew: Run for cover. Run and hide. I knew that as a five-year-
old. Had I lived a different life, getting thrown out of a speeding
minibus might have fazed me. I'd have stood there like an idiot,
going, "What's happening, Mom? Why are my legs so sore?"
But there was none of that. Mom said "Run," and I ran. Like the
gazelle runs from the lion, I ran.

We can think of our nervous system's regulation as an oven's ther-
mostat. We function best when we're in balance and not too hot or
too cold. But there are many situations that require us to turn the
heat up or down. In threatening environments, we want to notice and
feel our emotions more so they can help signal important information
and guide our behavior. When our emotional signals heat up to alert
us to a potential threat or loss of reward, we become more activated,
with louder body sensations, more alarming thoughts that match the
theme of the emotion, and urges to act in line with the emotion's message. If the perceived threat increases, we move further into fight-or-
flight mode, now burning so hot we won't miss the alarm.

Depending on how sensitive our alarm system is (based on our
unique biology and past adaptations) and how much practice we've
had in managing our emotions (such as with opportunities to learn
and practice emotional regulation skills from others), we can move
into high levels of activation while still being regulated. For example,
we can be very hot with anger but still use it in a skillful way. As
Aristotle said, "Anybody can become angry—that is easy; but to be
angry with the right person, and to the right degree, and at the right
time, and for the right purpose, and in the right way—that is not."

Some therapists name this range of emotional intensity that we can hold while still staying regulated the *zone of workability* or *window of tolerance.*

Our fight-or-flight mode is activated by our sympathetic nervous system (SNS) pumping adrenaline throughout our bodies, revving our heart rates, breathing, and blood flow to our muscles. Many of us end up with headaches; back, neck, chest, and shoulder pain from this muscle tension; and gastrointestinal upset from the blood moving away from digestion to focus on more urgent matters. As the SNS dilates our pupils, we may notice blurred vision. We can also feel dizzy, tingly, or short of breath.

When we move out of our zone of workability, we become activated in a dysregulated way. In this overheated zone, our blood flow leaves the higher brain's prefrontal cortex, which is slow and less useful in emergencies, in favor of our limbic system. This lower limbic road might not be as accurate in its assessments of the situation as the prefrontal cortex, but it works fast and intensely, exactly what we need to jump out of a car or fight off a predator. In this state, it can be challenging to think clearly, connect to our internal experience, or practice compassion and empathy. When someone asks us what's going on inside, we often have no clue and no words available to describe it.

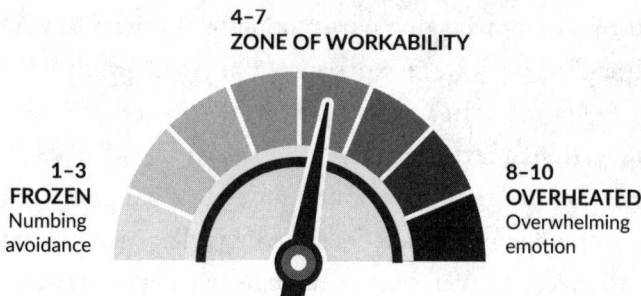

4–7
ZONE OF WORKABILITY

1–3
FROZEN
Numbing
avoidance

8–10
OVERHEATED
Overwhelming
emotion

Dial of Emotional Activation

When we experience a stress that's too intense, or we've been in fight-or-flight for too long, we may short-circuit into freeze, numbing or shutting down our feelings and sometimes even our behaviors. It's natural to avoid pain, so we may distract ourselves with activities or armor up with defenses to prevent us from feeling the overwhelming emotion (such as denying reality or our reactions to it, intellectualizing or joking instead of feeling, focusing only outward while ignoring our own experience, or compartmentalizing or dissociating so we don't access the painful feelings). This freeze response is protective by helping us push through and survive unrewarding environments or overwhelming stress. However, being in this state for too long or too often can make us feel emotionally and physically numb. We end up disconnected from others and from the emotion's important information about what we need, want, and care about.

The more activated or shut down we become with stress, the more we lose access to our higher brain and the harder it becomes to notice what's happening within us. Luckily, states of over- or underactivation are fully embodied with signature body sensations and action urges. We can learn to observe and track our bodies and urges to help us know what state we're operating from, as Ham supported Foo to do in therapy. We can also create a culture of connection where our loved ones also speak this language and can help us identify these states without judgment so we can help each other feel safe and co-regulate back into balance.

A core skill to managing our emotions is the practice of noticing and befriending what we're experiencing internally while we're experiencing it—or soon after, as we try to make sense of why we just shot off that mortifying text message.

We can learn our own signatures for each of our protective superheroes by observing and then documenting what we notice when we enter these states. We can start by noticing what our typical balanced, fight, flight, and freeze states feel and look like. Over the course of a week, we can practice paying attention to when we're emotionally

balanced, activated, or shut down and write down what our own responses looks like. For each category, we can ask ourselves the following questions:

> - BODY SENSATIONS: What do you feel in your body as you scan
>   the different parts?
>   □ What's the temperature of different areas?
>   □ What areas feel more tight or more loose?
>   □ What areas feel more heavy or more light?
>   □ Is there any movement in any areas, such as shaking, pulsing,
>   tingling?
>
> - ACTION URGES: Does it feel like your body is being pushed to act
>   in any certain way or adopt a certain posture, tone of voice, or
>   facial expression?
>
> - AUTOMATIC THOUGHTS: What do you believe about yourself
>   (such as your worth or ability to cope), others, the world?

RECOGNIZING COMMON TRIGGERS

As we explore our stress signatures, we may notice common triggers
that push us into these states. Sometimes, a trigger is what we see
at face value. For example, if we've struggled with an addiction, we
might notice that seeing the thing we're addicted to is a trigger. Or if
we have experienced violence, someone raising their voice or showing
obvious displays of hostility are likely triggers.

However, sometimes our triggers are more subtle. If we have experienced trauma in our lives or the group that we identify with has
historically or collectively faced oppression, we might unconsciously
be triggered by moments of power imbalances, such as when a bouncer
decides who gets admitted into a nightclub, or a teacher, disability
company, doctor, or boss exercises authority. Sometimes, the anger is

helpful and alerts us to harmful structures or behaviors in others that need changing, such as the activation that racialized people feel when facing police officers in the context of the well-documented harms of police brutality. And as always, we have many false alarms that speak more to the safety of our past, rather than the present, environment.

When we build awareness of our common triggers, they don't feel as personal or confusing when they arise. Instead, they can become predictable and lose their power over us. When we name—*Oh, that's my power imbalance trigger. Thanks, brain, for keeping me safe*—we can explore whether its message is warning us of a present or past threat and then move forward in the most helpful way.

STRATEGIES TO RETURN TO BALANCE

The first step to emotional regulation is to seek safety. As our alarms signal problems that need solving, we can assess whether an alarm is accurate, indicating a present problem, or a false alarm, based on misinterpretation or past learning. Our alarms will keep sounding until we hear their messages. We will never feel better if we keep ignoring a problem that could be solved if we were to address it. When it's within our control, we can remove ourselves from the threat or work to solve the problem.

We can next validate our response by acknowledging that the alarm makes sense right now, even if it isn't comfortable. For example, when I feel grief or anxiety following unfavorable elections, I can tell myself that it makes sense that I'm activated. My body is trying to tell me that these issues are important and I can't give up on our fight for a just and sustainable world.

Some of the triggers that activate our stress states are encoded into our DNA from long ago, when the threats that could harm us were very different. Evolution is a very slow process, and our nervous systems haven't evolved fast enough to adapt to our modern world, so sensory experiences that were once predictive of danger, such as heights, loud sounds, or being pushed around in a busy subway, still activate our threat response. This means that even though we know shooting across the sky in an airplane is statistically safe, we still get activated when exposed to it.

As we deepen our understanding around our neurodiversity, with each of us having unique settings for sensory sensitivity, we can also pay attention to how our external environments, such as excessive noise, visual stimuli, smells, and crowds, impact us. I've noticed that I get quite activated every time I enter a loud, crowded space or listen to my kid's rambunctious play or music, simply from the sensory overload itself, even when the environment is joyful and safe. As I've begun to pay more attention to my nervous system's distress, I can notice when I get overstimulated and take sensory breaks, or dose and change these environments when needed.

The architecture firm Forte Building Science believes that everyone benefits from the design features that make facilities friendly to people with sensory sensitivities.[3] It's easier for those of us who fall on the more sensitive side of the continuum to know when sensory stressors are impacting our health. We're like the canary at a rock concert who wants to leave at halftime. But these sensory experiences impact those with quieter alarms, too. They just don't know it. Numerous studies show that noise pollution, for example, subtly pushes us into fight-or-flight, inflaming our health, whether we're aware of it or not. Much of our irritability may arise from the sensory experiences of our environments.

We can also work to balance out our negativity biases by broadening the lens of our attention. We can shift our awareness to our safety in our present physical environments, our sense of awe at how the nature around us manages to create the circle of life, our gratitude for how our bodies manage to function in all the ways they do, the kindness and support of those around us, or the spiritual or philosophical truths we ascribe to when considering the bigger picture. We can also anchor ourselves with reminders of our purpose, history, or values like compassion, courage, or connection.

Then, when we notice our activation moving into fight, flight, or freeze states, we can practice bringing it back to balance by engaging in techniques that oppose the sympathetic nervous system (SNS) by activating the relaxation response of the parasympathetic nervous system (PNS) instead. Here are some strategies we can try:

1. THE COLD FACE DUNK: We humans have an evolutionary dive response that allows us to survive under water long enough to spear fish or fall in love with mermaids. This response operates by activating the PNS to slow down our heart rate, blood pressure, and therefore our oxygen use while under water. We can bio-hack our body into this response by bending over, holding our breath, and applying cold to our faces for up to sixty seconds. The cold part is the most important, but the other two parts help, too. This is best accomplished by dunking our faces in a bowl of ice water, or applying an icepack, especially over our cheekbones. The recent fad of cold-water swimming also stimulates this PNS response; although, when the entire body submerges in cold water, we first jolt it into SNS activation; then as we stay in the water, our PNS response kicks in. These exercises affect our heart rate and blood pressure, so if you have any heart problems or health conditions that might not react well to such changes, check with a health-care professional before you try this.

2. INTENSE PHYSICAL ACTIVITY: Moving our body intensely, from exercising and dancing to stress cleaning, sex, or strenuous labor— whatever feels intense for you—can also activate the relaxation response and release endorphins, calming the nervous system.

3. ABDOMINAL BREATHING PRACTICES: A variety of breathing practices can engage the PNS. Our body stimulates the SNS when we inhale and the PNS when we exhale. We also engage the PNS more with slow, deep belly (known as abdominal or diaphragmatic) breaths instead of breathing from our chest. We can put one hand on the chest and

one on the belly and see which area moves the most with each breath. When we are activated into fight-or-flight, we tend to breathe quickly from the chest. Instead, we can practice breathing slowly from our diaphragm, the muscle in our abdomen that pulls the lungs open to bring in air. This may take practice if we've spent our life breathing from our chest. We can also practice paced breathing, where our exhale is much longer than our inhale, to stimulate the PNS. Even slowing our breath down or pausing between breaths can calm us.

NOTE: Sometimes, noticing the breath can make us more anxious, because we might fuel it with threatening thoughts like *I'm doing it wrong* or *I'm not getting enough air.* If this feels true for you, you may want to start with a different skill—especially if you are high on the dial of activation—until you gain more comfort with the breath.

We can also distract ourselves by moving our attention somewhere neutral, away from the external stressor or unhelpful ruminations about it, such as:

1. 5–4–3–2–1: (as discussed in the last chapter)
    • Notice five sights we can see.
    • Notice four sensations we can feel.
    • Notice three sounds we can hear.
    • Notice two scents we can smell.
    • Notice one flavor we can taste.

2. PROGRESSIVE MUSCLE RELAXATION: We can move out of our heads and into the body (if this feels like a safe place for you) to release the physical tension of our fight-or-flight activation, or reconnect us with our feeling bodies if we're in freeze. In a systematic way, we can bring our kind attention to each area of the body, tense each muscle group, hold, then release the tension. We can modify this in any way to meet our body where it's at in each moment.

A possible sequence could be:
- Head
- Face
- Neck
- Upper back and shoulders
- Arms and hands
- Lower back, buttocks, and abdomen
- Legs
- Feet

3. HEALTHY DISTRACTION: I'm specifying "healthy" distraction because we want to ensure we don't avoid life by spending hours watching cat videos. You really can overdo distraction, no matter how warm and fuzzy it makes you feel in the moment. So, I'm only recommending distraction as a short-term strategy to allow the wave of activation to pass through you without making it worse by stewing in it, trying to push it away, or acting on it in ways that might not help the big picture.

I used to distract from the stress of reality by escaping into engaging TV dramas, until I heard a podcast from psychologist Thema Bryant.[4] "If your idea of relaxing before you go to sleep is watching three episodes of *Law & Order*, I would encourage you to think about, *Why is trauma relaxing to me?* It's harm, crime, violation, and attacks," she said. "Is that what's going to soothe me into my bedtime?" She explained that we often do this because it's normal and familiar. So many of us grew up in such high-stress environments that we mistakenly view peace as fake or boring. She convinced me to trade in my crime series for *Top Chef*—although I still stress out when my favorite contestants undercook their rice.

Distraction is not a long-term solution and doesn't address the cause of the alarms going off. Its purpose is to get our brains online and bring our body systems back to balance so we're capable of solving the real problems that our screaming alarms are signaling.

GROUNDING IN OUR GLIMMERS

We often talk about triggers, experiences that push us into fight, flight, or freeze. But we can also pay attention to glimmers in our environments, what psychotherapist Deb Dana, in her Rhythm of Regulation trainings, defines as micro-moments of regulation that foster feelings of well-being. "A glimmer could be as simple as seeing a friendly face, hearing a soothing sound, or noting something in the environment that brings a smile," Dana explains. "They are personal to each of us and one person's glimmer may be another person's trigger."

Because of our negativity bias that focuses on survival, we tend to be hypervigilant of potential triggers while ignoring the many glimmers in our environments in each moment. We can work to bring more attention to these grounding glimmers as a practice that can then become our new autopilot. But we can't only focus on glimmers while suppressing the impact of triggers. This practice is not a form of toxic positivity, a way to always look on the bright side and disavow your distress. "What they are is a reminder that the nervous system is exquisitely able to hold both dysregulation and regulation," Dana explains. In a day, we can both observe and hold the moments of distress and the moments of safety, balance, and connection.

When we're triggered into a state of fight-or-flight, our nervous system becomes more hypervigilant to threats. In this state, our negativity bias becomes more profound and our lens of awareness tunnel-visions on potential triggers, ignoring the glimmers that are present in the moment and outside of our narrow focus. When we notice we're tunnel-visioning in this way, we enhance our sense of safety by widening our spotlight of awareness to notice the glimmers of safety and connection in our present experience. While this may not solve the problem of the threat, it resources us by helping our nervous systems regulate toward a place of balance.

Considering all our senses, we can observe if there are any glimmers that bring on a feeling of balance, safety, or connection:

GROUNDING WITH GRATITUDE IN EVERYDAY GLIMMERS PRACTICE

We can begin practicing this skill regularly by setting an alarm at specific intervals or tying it to frequently occurring activities, such as every time we get a text or email, walk through a door, wash our hands, or eat or drink, to promote balance throughout the day. We can then apply this practice when we're noticing ourselves getting activated or deactivated to help us develop a sense of balance in these hard moments. I've added a gratitude practice to this exercise, but if it makes it too complicated, feel free to ignore the added step and stick with simply noticing glimmers.

- **EXTERNAL SENSES:**
  - See: Notice anything you can see that grounds you to a sense of safety, connection, or balance.
  - Hear: Notice anything you can hear that grounds you to a sense of safety, connection, or balance.
  - Touch: Notice anything you can touch that grounds you to a sense of safety, connection, or balance.
  - Smell: Notice anything you can smell that grounds you to a sense of safety, connection, or balance.
  - Taste: Notice anything you can taste that grounds you to a sense of safety, connection, or balance.
  - Can we extend gratitude to the miracle of how so many systems around us are functioning in balance, such as how our natural world with all its interdependent parts creates the rhythms of life with each tree, fly, and flower?

- **INTERNAL SENSES:**
  - Body Sensations: Notice anything you can feel in your body that grounds you to a sense of safety, connection, or balance.
  - Is there evidence that your body system is working as it should? For example, can you ground yourself in gratitude for functioning body systems or parts—that your respiratory, cardiac, skeletal, muscular, immune, digestive, hormonal, and nervous systems are functioning in the miracle of keeping you alive, even if they're noisy as they're doing their jobs?

- □ Is there evidence that your fight, flight, and freeze systems are working well to keep you safe?
- □ Mental Events: Notice any thoughts, associations, or memories in this moment that ground you to a sense of safety, connection, or balance.
- □ You can also practice bringing to mind a memory or thought that anchors you, such as a connection to a purpose, and practice gratitude for your capacity to have a mind system that can function in this way to help you.

- INTERCONNECTION: Can you notice any sense of connection to others or the natural or spiritual world that grounds you to a sense of safety, connection, or balance?
  - □ See if you can extend gratitude for these connections and the miracle of our synergy and interdependence.

- AWARENESS ITSELF: Can you notice your ability to be aware of all these things and see if this awareness can ground you in a sense of safety, connection, or balance?
  - □ Is there a way of framing everything you're aware of as not personal, permanent, or needing to be perfect? Can you extend gratitude to this awareness itself and how it can keep you grounded?

You may notice that some glimmers ground you best. Some of us may be more visual or auditory, while others might find focusing on our interconnection the most impactful. When we're in fight, flight, or freeze, it can be hard to remember to expand our attention to glimmers, so writing them down ahead of time can help. Next time, you'll have a list to try in those hard moments. You can list some glimmers that are especially grounding to you here:

_____

_____

_____

THE ABCs OF REGULATION

We can also work at the level of our subcortical brains to soothe our three-threat alarm systems of anger, fear, and separation distress with the ABCs we discussed in Chapter Three. You can explore what unique activities would restore your sense of agency, bonding, and containment using the space in each box to personalize your own strategies.

AGENCY	Engage in an activity that brings on a sense of mastery, autonomy, empowerment, or justice.
BONDING	Connect with supportive others and community, surround yourself with safe and regulated people, or engage in activities that give you a sense of belonging.
CONTAINMENT	Seek safety. Create a stable routine or ritual to anchor you, or move your attention to parts of your environment that feel safe, predictable, and secure.

We can also engage our subcortical reward systems of seeking, care, lust, and play, because such connecting, meaningful activities can move us out of our inflammatory threat networks, even when life is stressful. If we're anxious as a passenger in a car or bus after a motor vehicle accident, rather than allowing our thoughts to focus on all the potential threats of the commute, we can move our attention into our seeking system by working on a creative project or task. Similarly, after I had children, the situations that often made me anxious in the past no longer felt as activating because I had switched into my care networks by attending to my children's needs when they were with me. In the same way, when I'm supporting someone as a trauma therapist, despite being reminded of the true threats in the world around us for hours each day, because I'm engaging my seeking and care systems in the role of their therapist, I am able to stay regulated in the midst of the distress.

GROUNDING IN THE GLIMMERS OF LIGHT

In *The Light We Give*, human rights activist Simran Jeet Singh reckons with how to live as a Sikh man in the US, from growing up being bullied for wearing a turban in Texas, to facing daily racism with accusations of being a terrorist. The reality of terrorism in the US is that the majority of such acts in the past three decades have been perpetrated by white right-wing extremists, and mostly against racialized communities.[5] When one of these right-wing extremists attacked and killed innocent members of a Sikh community in their place of worship in Wisconsin, Singh felt both shocked and unsurprised. Yet as he spent time with the community, he observed a kind of resilience and emotional balance in the face of atrocity that he'd never before seen.

Every community member he spoke to referred to the Sikh teaching of *chardi kala*, a phrase that translates roughly to "everlasting optimism." Singh wrote, "Every day, as Sikhs pray for the uplifting of all humanity (*sarbat da bhala*), they speak of *chardi kala* in the same breath." *Chardi kala* became the community's slogan and was printed on shirts and used in fundraisers, providing "hope in the midst of crushing pain."

He also watched the community draw on the Sikh teachings of *seva,* which encourage many small acts of care toward our interconnected collective when facing injustices and suffering in the world. "On their own, single acts of *seva* might seem random, but taken together, they bring light into our world and into each of us," just like the light of one lantern inspires others to follow the same path, Singh explained. As others join in, the small and humble action of one ripples into a meaningful change for all.

When Singh spoke to a group of Sikh children about the massacre, they tried to make sense of how someone could cause so much harm to others, when they believe that everyone comes from and shares the same light. One of the girls spoke up, saying, "[The killer] didn't see that light in himself or in other people. That's why he could hurt them."

Living from our inherent light requires our nervous systems to be regulated. Our dysregulation into the depths of hate, panic, and apathy is contagious and easily hijacks our minds to go along with dynamics that hurt us all. But so is the brightness of compassion, connection, and hope. It might feel selfish to prioritize our own balance and light when the world is facing so much pain. But then we can offer the gentle light of our own equanimity and care to a world that so desperately needs to come back into balance.

Just as we're all vulnerable to being hijacked by dysregulation, we also have the power to help each other co-regulate and come back online, revealing the light in each of us, one person at a time. Sometimes, the most generous gift we can offer the world is to work to regulate our own nervous systems so we can help pull others back into balance with us.

SEVEN

GETTING OUT OF
OUR HEADS

Somewhere along the way we were taught to stop feeling
instead of being taught to stop what harms us, as though the
feeling were our enemy, as though the feeling were hurting us.
—PRENTIS HEMPHILL

I CHECKED MY GPS AGAIN. A LONG RED LINE ALERTED ME TO A TRAFFIC STANDSTILL,
seemingly the entire way to my retreat center. Already regretting my
decision to register for a week of silent meditation on embodied mindfulness, I thought back to my email confirmation. "Please ensure you
arrive promptly by 4 p.m.," it had said. "At that time, you will receive
important information before entering Noble Silence."

It was 1 p.m. The estimated time of arrival on my phone's map
was 4:12.

My car inched ahead.

The ETA changed: 4:15 p.m. *Shit.*

4:23 p.m.

I changed lanes, twice.

4:22 p.m.

I looked away from my GPS in relief. *I'm making time.*

4:27 p.m. Merging again. My body cringed. *I should have anticipated this delay. What will they think of me?* My hands shook as adrenaline shot flames into my cheeks. *What kind of person arrives flustered*

and late to a meditation retreat? The others will spot the imposter the mo-
ment I arrive. They will already be all solemn and silent, and I'll be left
with days of wondering who the hell all these people are and what are the
instructions.

I finally arrived. It was 4:58 p.m.

A DOZEN HUMBLE BUILDINGS SNUGGLED UP TO ACRES OF FERTILE HILLS, WITH
pockets of trees surrounding a few streams and a large pond. When
I entered the main building, a man sprang out of his seat, setting the
tone of this strange place with a massive smile.

"I'm so sorry," I said. "I got stuck in traffic. I should have—"

"Welcome!" he said. "And no worries. You're not the only one.
Lucky for you, all the work assignments have been taken, so you don't
have any chores this retreat. I will show you to your room and give
you a tour."

Relief swept over me, but it was unsettling: I lost faith in my own
assumptions. Keeping my pessimism unchallenged felt safer, more
predictable. Even if it was predictable in its misery.

Everyone had already entered Noble Silence. They instructed us
to avoid eye contact to offer everyone their space for silence without
intrusions. I entered the meditation hall, smiling and nodding to everyone I passed, then scolding myself afterward for breaking the rules.
I could handle the silence itself, but I needed to scan faces to monitor
for threats.

I found the last open spot, pleased to be hidden in the back corner,
and placed my meditation cushion on the floor. *For a group that prides*
itself on nonattachment, they sure do hoard pillows.

As I sat down, a part of me felt stoic and strong, a minimalist
aching my way to enlightenment. My knee burned and my left foot
tingled. The chairs on the side seduced me with their back support, but
I tensed my shoulders and crossed my legs the other way, then back
again, but only when no one was looking.

Other meditators glided in, each bowing toward the front as they entered. *Oh shit. I didn't bow.* I watched each bow, trying to perfect it in my mind. Some held their hands together over their face with a subtle nod; others flaunted their flexibility by bowing deeper and bigger than the person before. I couldn't decide how I should bow. Or should I bow? Is it cultural appropriation if I do? Or lack of respect if I don't? Maybe I will just come early each time so no one sees me.

I noticed the teacher at the front in a flowered dress and cardigan, all in muted pastels. It seemed an odd choice—not the solemn robes of other teachers, but also not a fierce statement either. She seemed submissive, passive, even fragile. My body deflated watching her. She was not the role model I craved.

But then she sat down in a chair. A chair! No masochistic leg pretzels. This seemed defiant, energizing my mind. Maybe she was the Joni Mitchell of meditation teachers: a hero in her noncompliance to the scene.

Joni closed her eyes, and without instruction, we all just sat.

I looked around, distracted by a fly bouncing about on the other side of the room, ramming his head against the window. I felt for the little guy, so able to see the light on the other side but unable to figure out how to get there. He tried harder, buzzing louder. I wanted to swat him out of his misery, but then felt instant guilt for betraying the Buddhist teachings of honoring all living beings within the first hour of my arrival.

I noticed the woman next to me, her back muscles twitching as she sat, like they were trying to let me know that she, too, had her demons. I felt a softening toward her as she shifted about, repositioning her pillows again and again. Maybe she will be my friend.

The gong echoed through the meditation hall, and Joni stepped, painfully slowly, toward the door, quoting meditation teacher Thich Nhat Hanh's "walking as if you are kissing the Earth with your feet." The sincere faces of my fellow meditators didn't help, as each got up and followed Joni on her trip, as we waited for her to levitate.

"Simply noticing the physical sensations of your body walking, the anchor to your present-moment experience . . ."

"Arriving in the life that's right here . . ."

"Lifting . . . swinging . . . placing . . ."

The group funneled out like a zombie apocalypse on drugs while the bagpipes of my mind blared as I, too, lifted and swung with precision, picturing them all dancing in unison to Michael Jackson's "Thriller," as I moved my hips to the beat.

Damn. Thinking, thinking.

LIFTING . . . SWINGING . . . PLACING . . .

LIFTING . . . SWINGING . . . PLACING . . .

I LONGED FOR THE GONG TO GIVE ME PERMISSION TO END EACH MEDITATION, ANTICIPATing the liberation in just a few more moments. But with each metallic roar thrust onto the silence of the group, I rejoiced only for a brief moment before realizing that it instructed me to start the next meditation.

Sitting meditation.

Walking meditation.

Sitting meditation.

Eating meditation.

Sitting meditation.

Walking meditation.

Sitting meditation.

Eating meditation.

I COULDN'T WAIT FOR THE DAY TO BE OVER, BUT AS I BURROWED INTO MY BLANKETS, sleep tantalized me, forever out of reach. While my body submitted willingly to the bed, my mind eagerly hunted the past and future, reliving heartbreaks and forecasting disaster.

I tried to get out of bed unnoticed, timing my movements to the crescendos of the snores surrounding me, fearing that I had broken the rules of spiritual enlightenment by having insomnia. The floor squeaked, making each undetected step a celebrated victory, as if I were escaping a lifelong system of shoulds and should nots.

Outside, the darkness disappointed me, although I wasn't sure what else I expected, perhaps radiant lights and purple clouds announcing my entry into nirvana?

The lights were on in the cafeteria, so I slid into the building. I rushed to the corner when I discovered a blessed toast station, with jars of peanut butter and jam perched on their pedestal to soothe all the night's woes. For some reason, I felt relief, as if the toast station proved that midnight peanut butter cravings were a universal side effect of meditation, or being human. I looked up and saw Joni sitting there, toast in hand. She met my eyes and I caught a glimpse of her smile before I forced my eyes back to my feet and scurried back to bed.

SITTING.

Walking.
Sitting.
Eating.
Sitting.
Walking.
Sitting.
Eating.
Trapped.
Tension in my hands.
Tightness in my chest.
Sadness in my throat.
Heaviness in my eyes.

Tears.

Shaky hands.

Sweaty palms.

I STOOD OUTSIDE JONI'S DOOR, AS IF I WERE WAITING IN THE PRINCIPAL'S OFFICE.

Joni opened the door, her gentle presence immediately inter-rupting all the images in my mind of my banishment from this vol-untary jail.

"How is your experience of this retreat?"

"Fine," I said.

Joni nodded, her patient silence inviting more than any line of questioning could.

"I'm not good enough," I said. "I've been cheating. I sneak away during the walking meditations and wander the trails, looking at trees. I sleep through the morning meditations and do yoga in the field when everyone is doing their chores. I'm up walking around in the middle of the night and can't figure out how to close doors quietly. I just can't do this right."

Joni placed her hand on her heart as she spoke. "Oh, hon, that's quite a storm of harsh thoughts passing through. I wonder if we can pause for a moment to be with this. What feelings arise as you sit here now?"

"Frustration . . . fear . . ." I threw at her without thinking.

"And how do you experience this in your body?"

"Heaviness under my eyes, over my heart. Tension in my throat."

Tears arrived.

Joni moved her hand in small circles over her heart.

"And maybe there's another feeling underneath?"

I looked right into Joni's eyes and knew I didn't need to name it.

"Can we invite this sadness in, too? Meet it at the door, smiling? It seems to me that this is exactly what you've been needing to so tenderly hold in this retreat," she said. "My body fills with delight picturing you in the forest with the trees, doing yoga in the grass, sleeping when you need to sleep. The schedule here is a suggestion, but we each have our own path. The true practice is to be flexible, paying attention to whatever our body needs in each new moment, truly feeling our bodies, not just thinking about them, so we can learn how to best nurture ourselves. Mindfulness is not just what we do, but how we do it. How can we inhabit our own bodies gently and cultivate kindness toward our own experiences?"

THE DOMINANCE OF THINKING

When we start to observe where our attention spends most of its time, we often find that we live in our heads, far away from our bodies, especially those of us from more colonial cultures or who live with trauma, depression, or anxiety.

While I fell into psychiatry on a whim, having gone to medical school with plans of working abroad for Doctors Without Borders, when looking back, I see early hints of how I ended up on this path. In my youth, I obsessively read books that I'd chosen for their stream-of-consciousness techniques, such as the works of Toni Morrison, Virginia Woolf, and Franz Kafka.

Let me be clear: I was not the hip artsy type in college who sat at back tables of smoky bars discussing literature, philosophy, and politics, as much as I wish this were true. I wore a lot of sweatpants, majored in kinesiology and health promotion, and spent all my time working as a lifeguard and fitness instructor, while hanging out with my jock classmates, who also wore a lot of sweatpants. But I spent the spaces in between as a closeted introvert, reading on breaks or listening to audiobooks during chores and workouts, and these authors became some of my coolest imaginary friends.

We can trace stream of consciousness back to Buddhism's early texts, with the concept of *citta-santāna*, translated from Sanskrit to mean "mindstream." It describes our moment-to-moment awareness of all our sensory perceptions and mental events, as we learned in Chapter Six. When novelists use this technique in their writing, we

get a true taste of living in someone else's messy head and body, beyond the logical, edited versions that we tend to see in thoughtfully
constructed stories. It's voyeurism at its best—at least when you love
humans as much as I do.

When reading the works of stream of consciousness by authors
from colonial cultures like my own, we can see that so much of the
content is focused on thoughts rather than feelings, and especially
not how feelings are experienced in our bodies. Thoughts are easy
to spot, seem rational, and occupy much of our conscious awareness.
Emotional reactions are far more of an enigma, fusing signals from
threats and rewards in our present environment with reactions to un-
clear triggers linked to past wounds, all happening largely outside of
our awareness. Without practice, most of us aren't aware of what emotions we're feeling most of the time.

A few years ago, I joined a white settler community of learning to
explore anti-racism, struggling together to become more conscious of
how the dynamics of racism show up in our own lives and communities.
While cultural humility training often seeks to understand the cultures
of marginalized groups, we frequently miss out on reflecting on our own
unconscious conditioning as members of the dominant colonial culture
of white supremecy that created and perpetuates racism.

While we've all explicitly learned that racism is bad, we also implicitly learn certain racist emotional reactions, beliefs, and habits
without any conscious awareness of them. Resmaa Menakem explains
that we've focused our anti-racism efforts in the wrong direction by
following the same failed strategy of letting our explicit thinking
minds dominate. "For the past three decades, we've earnestly tried
to address white-body supremacy in America with reason, principles,
and ideas—using dialogue, forums, discussions, education, and mental
training," he wrote. "But the widespread destruction of Black bodies
continues. We've tried to teach our brains to think better about race.
But white-body supremacy doesn't live in our thinking brains. It lives
and breathes in our bodies."[1]

For example, when a person who's racialized as white sees a person who racialized as Black, they may be activated into fight-or-flight as an implicit emotional reaction based on unconscious learning and modeling from their dominant culture. While those from marginalized racial groups cannot be racist toward those who oppress them, since racism and abuse require the dominance of power, they can still implicitly learn messages about race. For instance, despite explicitly wanting to express valid anger in a situation, many BIPOC people may implicitly learn to fear or fawn instead, both from intergenerational and personal conditioning, to unconsciously protect themselves from white supremacy's enduring pattern of harm. In both these situations, we can throw a lot of second arrows of guilt, shame, or confusion when our emotional reactions don't align with our explicit beliefs (or even make conscious sense to us).

Ruth King, a mindfulness teacher and diversity consultant who wrote *Mindful of Race*, explores how our implicit patterns of racial learning are often outside of our awareness. Because white folks aren't marginalized for our group identity, our racial positioning as white isn't often in our awareness as it is for those who face daily oppression because of their racial group identity. Rather than recognize how we uniquely experience the world through our own racial group conditioning, we unconsciously may assume that whiteness is neutral (and not a diverse identity with its own culture). Instead, white folks often focus only on our individual identities and merits. It's easy to "not see race," believe that a country isn't racist, or deny the need for diversity, equity, and inclusivity in our organizations when we're in the dominant group who benefits from racism.

Ruth King encourages racial affinity groups as a way of "coming together as white people and tenderly examining this thing called whiteness that other races seem to know about" as a crucial link in racial healing and harmony. In my community of support, we explored our own conditioning as white settlers that we often overlook, based on Kenneth Jones and Tema Okun's *Dismantling Racism* work, such as our emotional habits of prioritizing thoughts over feelings, the written word over other ways of knowing, and comfort over growth.[2]

We're not alone. Many Western philosophers and psychologists alike hoped we could explicitly think our way into an easier existence. French philosopher René Descartes captured the sentiment clearly, arguing, "I think, therefore I am," paving the way for the cognitive part of cognitive behavioral therapy's (CBT) approach of trying to change how we feel by changing our thoughts. Other kinds of therapy also focus on explicit learning, such as building insight, challenging unhelpful thinking, and rational problem-solving (and I will spend an entire chapter on exploring how to work with thoughts later). But I'm intentionally not offering that chapter first, especially since many of you, like me, may have been conditioned by cultures where thinking dominates over feeling, and where we're more focused on the explicit content of thoughts and conversations than the implicit process of how we feel and relate to them.

The biggest problem with this thinking-dominant approach is that when we're distressed and reaching for strategies to feel better, we're often in fight, flight, or freeze states. Or we're in a state of depression or anxiety, where our emotions are giving birth to a lot of pessimistic and catastrophic thoughts. In these states, our thoughts keep circling the drain to nowhere productive, just as you observed in my first meditation retreat, except to give us evidence that we're in a stressed state. At these times, the content of our thoughts is more a symptom of the emotional state we are in than an accurate readout of reality. And as you remember, we don't have access to the higher parts of our brain in these stressed states, so thinking approaches aren't very useful. It sounds great when you're cozied up in the safety of your bed or therapist's couch, but very hard to practice when your implicit learning from past threats just hijacked your brain and punted you into a stress response.

Another challenge is that when we think, we can travel to the past and future, experiencing these different times' alarms in our bodies as if they are happening in the present. We relive past adversities and potential catastrophes over and over in our bodies, moving us into a matching stress response, magnifying our suffering.

After spending the first three decades of my life stuck in my head, trying to rationally think my way out of my pain with little success, I've now learned to shift my awareness to my embodied feelings instead. And I can attest it's much more comfortable, even when we're focusing right in on the distressing sensations in the present.

When we move our attention out of our heads and into our bodies, our relationship with all these alarms ends up being a mere unmemorable fling instead of a drawn-out and agonizing affair, where every one of our friends curse each time we bring it up in looping repetition. Instead, when our alarms are felt in the body, without overthinking them or needing to push them away, we can ride the waves quite effortlessly, making our alarms neither scary nor intolerable.

ACT therapist Russ Harris offers the analogy of a hotel to illustrate this strategy. We have no control over who arrives in the lobby. We can notice when a thought has entered, maybe even flirt a bit to see if it has any endearing qualities, but we don't have to invite them upstairs, especially if they're setting off all our alarms. Instead, we have the power to choose which thoughts we spend time entertaining. We can chat up a worry thought about a future earthquake enough to ensure our home is prepared with emergency supplies if the event were to occur, but once we've learned all we can from the conversation, we don't need to repeat the same conversation again and again. Instead, we can use our kind attention skills to notice the loop and then change the channel of our awareness to other things. If the thought won't get the picture and leave us alone, we can move our awareness to a less stressful object of attention—the body, which is always available to us and anchored strongly to the present.

If we experience trauma, which is often stored in the body, the body may not be a safe place to begin our practice. Many people describe the body as the least safe place to inhabit, since it can feel so strongly anchored to traumatic memories of the past. Depending on the intensity of our trauma, it can take years of healing work to build a sense of comfort and safety in being with our own body sensations. If this is true for you, try beginning with the external senses of hearing, vision, touch, smell, and taste, and then notice more neutral areas of the body first, such as the feet and hands. Then we can slowly build up our comfort in experiencing other body sensations, often with the help of a professional trained in trauma therapy.

The health of all our systems, including our bodies and nervous systems, requires all our parts to be in balance, without allowing any one part, like thinking, to dominate over the others. I'm not suggesting that we don't think. Rather, we want to integrate our thinking brains with our feeling bodies so that they communicate, work together, and share the spotlight. One of my teachers once explained this balance as the goal of psychotherapy: we learn to think while feeling and feel while thinking. We also want to balance our focus on our inner and outer worlds, so no part of our system is neglected.

SURFING DISCOMFORT IN THE BODY

Toni Morrison's novels taught me to feel in my body in a way that had never been modeled to me. Decades before her vivid prose resuscitated our hearts with both visceral and symbolic depth, she was a graduate student studying the authors who first brought stream of consciousness to the mainstream. She argued in her thesis that the defining feature of contemporary Western literature—and its tragic flaw—is the "widespread concept of man as a thing apart—as an individual who, if not lost, is impressively alone." These writers revealed how Western culture suffered from a disconnection not only from others, but also from our own feeling bodies. We connect to others through our feelings. As we sever our connection to this part of ourselves, we also lose our lifelines to each other.

Often, we repress our feelings as an automatic habit to avoid emotional pain, especially when we've been conditioned to fear it. For example, in William Faulkner's novel *As I Lay Dying*, as the protagonist's mother is taking her last breaths of life, rather than connecting to the feelings of grief in his body, he diverts his attention to his stream of thoughts, ruminating about his half-brother who's building the casket outside her window:

> Because I said if you wouldn't keep on sawing and nailing at it
> until a man can't sleep even and her hands laying on the quilt
> like two of them roots dug up and tried to wash and you couldn't
> get them clean. I can see the fan and Dewey Dell's arm. I said if
> you'd just let her alone. Sawing and knocking, and keeping the air
> always moving so fast on her face that when you're tired you can't
> breathe it, and that goddamn adze going One lick less. One lick
> less. One lick less until everybody that passes in the road will have
> to stop and see it and say what a fine carpenter he is.

Keeping our awareness stuck on thoughts like this, instead of directly feeling the pain of the present, only prolongs the pain by reactivating the feelings over and over without ever processing them. We end up continuously displacing or running away from the discomfort without holding it in awareness long enough to feel and digest it. We then need to constantly exert effort to keep these feelings at arm's length, as if forever trying to push a beach ball under water. Eventually, we will tire, and the ball will pop up and hit us with an even greater force than if we'd allowed it to float on the surface all along.

When we're anxious or depressed, functional MRI scans show that part of our default mode network—the neural system tasked with thinking about oneself in past and future and in relation to others—becomes overactive when we face negative events.[3, 4] It's why depression and anxiety are conditions of being lost in our heads with rumination and worry. You'd guess that moving our attention away from the distressing feelings and body sensations would make us feel less pain. But the more the default network dominates, the more intensely we're acti-

vated into distress, even though we aren't consciously aware of the activated feelings in our bodies. The default mode causes us to amplify the
distress by both identifying personally with circumstances and time-
traveling to threats of the past or future. And this all typically happens
outside our awareness, so we don't even notice that we're dysregulating
until it's too late.[5] Trying to escape our embodied feelings by thinking
our way out of them only makes them hit us harder.

We can also voluntarily suppress our emotions. Many of us doctors and therapists were trained to do this, puffing into the defense of
our thinking-dominant expertise on a subject, analyzing and spewing
facts from the comfort of our presumably unaffected position. But
no amount of book learning will make us invincible to the pain of
being human, nor will being "professional" and "neutral" by avoiding feelings—and thus our ability to connect as a human—help our
patients. We can't explore a patient's emotions and defenses under the
false guise of "objectivity" while pretending we're not also in the ring
bouncing about with them. Instead, we need to be curious about the
automatic alarms and assumptions of all the players involved, and that
includes how we participate in each dynamic.

Others can also force or condition us to disconnect from our feelings, as we discussed earlier when we talked about the political pris-
oners of the Khmer Rouge. Political organizer and somatic therapist
Prentis Hemphill explains how emotions become enslaved whenever
bodies are oppressed in *What It Takes to Heal: How Transforming Ourselves Can Change the World*:

> For our ancestors, certain emotions and expressions of those
> emotions were forbidden in public because they might give rise
> to an energy willing and capable of opposing injustice. To violate
> that unwritten order was to risk more violence. . . . There is a
> danger in expressing emotion, too, because of what it might do
> to those training to be the oppressor. Hearing the familiar and
> heartrending cry of a human in pain could threaten to interrupt the

project of making socially acceptable that which was inhumane. Closing off their ears and hearts to such a sound meant learning to extinguish their empathy, to teach a narrow compassion to their children, and to find a tenuous, anxious safety in pretending the human they hurt was a monster. Empathy, mutuality, and connection are dangerous to injustice. They can unravel what is otherwise a fragile, imposed order. For safety reasons, then, we are all taught to push our emotions down and away rather than to feel them. If we felt, imagine what we might change.

Toni Morrison's writing was a bold rebellion against this silencing of emotions on all sides of our systems of oppression. It wasn't until fifteen years into her career of teaching university English and working as the first Black senior editor for Random House's fiction department that she published her first novel, *The Bluest Eye,* a book *The New York Times* praised as "so charged with pain and wonder that the novel becomes poetry."[6] She later explained, "If there's a book that you want to read, but it hasn't been written yet, then you must write it." Morrison wrote what we all needed to read: words that reawakened our feelings. And in doing so, she helped heal our alienation from both our own bodies and each other.

IF YOU CAN FEEL IT, YOU CAN HEAL IT

When we ignore our emotional alarms, whether they're unconsciously repressed, intentionally suppressed, or involuntarily oppressed, our alarm systems must ring even louder to be heard. While it might seem counterintuitive, moving our attention to the direct body sensations and feelings of our alarms allows them to quiet. They no longer need to keep signaling their distress because we've received their message.

When we catch ourselves stuck in our heads while ignoring our feelings, we can pause to notice how this focus on the content of our thoughts is dominating our attention. Then we can take a step back from the content of our thoughts and instead notice the process of how we are stuck in our thoughts, such as with ruminating or worrying. We can bring our attention back into balance by focusing on our body sensations—or if that feels too unsafe at the beginning, our external senses of touch, taste, smell, hearing, sight, or our sense of connection to others, nature, spirituality, or even awareness itself. Shifting our attention in this way can be quite grounding, because thoughts often feel anchorless and disorganized, jumping between different times, abstractions, and associations, while our other senses offer a more concrete, steady anchor to the present moment.

Observing our embodied feelings is surprisingly more comfortable than the mental distress of trying to think about or avoid them. Our emotions impact us more intensely when we aren't explicitly aware of them. When we bring our embodied feelings into awareness, we regain the power to work with them effectively.

We can observe the process of avoiding or thinking about emotions instead of feeling them. For example, Faulkner's protagonist could notice he's stuck in thinking dominance and be curious as to what he's feeling in that moment. He may notice a shaky sense of fear and tension in his body, or perhaps a heaviness of grief in his chest and throat. He may then become aware of how much he fears feeling these things, as he's implicitly learned from his past or culture that he can't stand vulnerable emotions. He may realize that this fear is an old false alarm that's bullying him into running away from feelings that he's actually quite capable of holding. Instead, he can move his focus into his body, exploring these sensations in the present moment.

"If you surrender to the wind, you can ride it," Toni Morrison wrote in *Song of Solomon*. The same is true for surrendering to waves of feelings, especially if we sense them in a specific way: with acceptance and curiosity about whatever arises, without adding the extra suffering of making it personal, evaluating it as bad or permanent, or striving for it to be different than it already is. We can remind ourselves of the three insights of mindfulness, as summarized by Ruth King: nothing is perfect, permanent, or personal.

ANCHORING IN BODY SENSATIONS

This exercise is based on Buddhism's four qualities of body sensations described by the four elements (earth/solidity, water/tension, fire/temperature, and air/movement).

1. **PAUSE TO BRING KIND AWARENESS TO YOUR INTERNAL PROCESS: WHERE AM I ON THE DIAL OF ACTIVATION?**

   If you notice you're over- or underactivated outside your zone of tolerance/workability, try practicing some of the skills from the last chapter or seek out co-regulation from others to help bring your activation into a more helpful place.

2. **WHERE'S YOUR ATTENTION FOCUSED RIGHT NOW? IS THINKING MODE DOMINATING?**

   How helpful is it to focus on thinking right now? How much are your thoughts fueling your activation or distracting you from feeling what needs to be felt?

3. **CAN YOU MOVE YOUR ATTENTION TO THE BODY SENSATIONS PRESENT RIGHT NOW?**

   A. Notice the temperature in different areas of your body.

   B. Notice how heavy or light the different areas feel.

   C. Notice how tense or loose the different areas feel.

   D. Notice the unique sensations of movement or stillness in different parts.

4. **NOTICE YOUR REACTIONS OF PERSONALIZING, JUDGING THE SENSATIONS AS GOOD OR BAD, OR WANTING TO CLING TO OR PUSH THEM AWAY.**

   See if you can bring a kind attention to these reactions themselves, also allowing all the body sensations of these reactions to be here, too. How do these reactions feel in the body?

   ☐ Notice the temperature in the different areas of the body.
   ☐ Notice how heavy or light the different areas feel.
   ☐ Notice how tense or loose the different areas feel.

□   Notice the unique sensations of movement or stillness in
     different parts.

5. EACH TIME YOU NOTICE A NEW THOUGHT OR REACTION ARISE IN RESPONSE TO
THESE BODY SENSATIONS, KEEP BRINGING THIS KIND AND CURIOUS ATTENTION
BACK TO THE BODY, OVER AND OVER, ALLOWING ALL THE INNER EXPERIENCES TO
BE HERE JUST AS THEY ARE, AS IF YOU'RE GENTLY AND PATIENTLY TRAINING A
PUPPY TO HEEL.

It's often the thoughts and reactions that arise to feelings and body sensations that make them so unpleasant, not the sensations themselves. I remember I once received a message that brought up a lot of shame right before hopping into my car for a long drive. Stuck seat-belted into that small metal box with no way of discharging the emotion in my usual ways of cuddling a loved one or moving my body, I decided to practice what I teach in my mindfulness classes.

I scanned my body for temperature, noticing the warmth flushing in my cheeks, chest, and upper arms, and the coldness in my hands. I realized how the heat and cold felt quite neutral and impersonal; they were simply passing noisy body sensations when stripped of my identification and interpretations of them. I observed my chest, jaw, and hands tightening as my heart region felt heavy. Again, I realized the sensations themselves all felt quite tolerable and impersonal. I scanned for movement, noticing my heart racing and my arms and lips tingling. It just felt like the impersonal, imperfect, and impermanent movements of muscles and nerves.

In *The Bluest Eye*, Toni Morrison wrote, "You looked at them and wondered why they were so ugly; you looked closely and could not find the source. Then you realized that it came from conviction, their conviction. It was as though some mysterious all-knowing master had given each one a cloak of ugliness to wear, and they had each accepted it without question." Morrison is referring to how we've created the concept of race and assigned it an imaginary value based solely on how we've been conditioned to interpret it.

In the same way, we've spent so much effort trying to rid ourselves of our "ugly" feelings that we often don't even realize that what we're running away from is its ugly cloak of conviction that makes us believe they are bad. Instead, we can see feelings for what they are underneath: dances of impersonal, impermanent, and noisy body sensations designed to help us navigate the rewards and threats of the world to keep our systems in balance. Our feelings aren't what's threatening or rewarding. They are alerting us to what's threatening or rewarding. When we spend all of our effort focused on ridding ourselves of the alarms without addressing the problems they're signaling, they will keep sounding louder and louder until we receive their messages.

We're not alone in fearing these sensations. We internalize many ways of avoiding or displacing emotions from our families and wider cultures, just like I've implicitly learned to prioritize thinking over feeling. My training as a physician within our thinking-dominant medical culture only further entrenched this defense.

So many of us get trapped in anxious and depressive cycles because our conditioning of thinking dominance perpetuates our distress. When healthy emotional alarms of fear, shame, guilt, anger, grief, or low mood arise, we may add second arrows of thinking that they shouldn't be there. We ruminate about why we're feeling so bad, assume we should be feeling better, hunt for causes based on our past mistakes, and worry that this feeling will last forever.

When I gave myself permission for a low mood or burnout to be here, these passing experiences stopped escalating into depression from all the second arrows that fueled my distress. I learned to notice when I got caught up in thoughts of trying to figure out what was wrong with me for feeling so down or worrying about how this current state would affect my future functioning. I could then label the process of being stuck in thoughts about my emotional state instead of feeling it and move my attention back into balance by sensing my body and the world around me. While it felt unnatural at first—and required a lot of effort at the beginning to create a new habit—over time, it has become my new autopilot, ensuring my system stays in balance.

WHEN THE DEFENSE HURTS MORE THAN THE FEELING

We defend against the ugly cloaks we associate with feelings in a wide variety of ways. Freud first proposed the concept of defense mechanisms to describe the adaptive strategies we employ to protect us from unwanted emotions that may overwhelm us. They allow us to function in the short term in the face of stress. However, like with everything else, when we get stuck rigidly using one strategy, our mental health suffers. Instead, we are healthiest when flexibly using a variety of defenses for temporary relief. We want to be aware of when we've armored up in a defense mechanism and then be able to take that armor off again when it's no longer helpful.

For example, when I worked in the emergency or surgical room, I armored up by compartmentalizing and suppressing my fear, grief, or anger so I could focus on the tasks of the medical emergencies in front of me. I also needed to take this armor off when talking to patients and families, or when I returned home after a shift. If I remained rigidly stuck in this defense all the time, I'd lose my capacity to attune to the emotional needs of others, learn from the essential information that my emotions were signaling to me, and communicate these needs to others.

Here are some common defense mechanisms that we all may use at times:

- DENIAL: We avoid accepting our painful realities and their associated emotions, such as blocking out our grief after we've lost someone important to us or our fear from the threatening reality of climate change.

- **DISSOCIATION**: We split off and detach from parts of our experience, such as detaching from our emotional experience, memory of a traumatic event, or awareness of our external reality.
- **REPRESSION**: Rather than acknowledging the existence of unwanted emotions, memories, thoughts, and urges, we unconscously push them down or split them off from our awareness.
- **SUPPRESSION**: The same as repression but done consciously, with awareness.
- **PROJECTION**: Instead of acknowledging unwanted emotions, thoughts, or urges in ourselves, we project them onto others and tell ourselves that the unwanted inner experiences are theirs instead of our own.
- **DISPLACEMENT**: Instead of feeling unwanted emotions, we misplace them onto other people or objects that don't feel as threatening. For example, rather than feeling angry with a boss who has the power to fire us, we get angry with our family or partner instead.
- **RATIONALIZATION/INTELLECTUALIZATION**: Rather than feeling the unwanted emotion, we split off the emotional component and only think about the situation.
- **COMPARTMENTALIZATION**: We split off unwanted emotions and their associated thoughts, memories, body sensations, and urges from other parts of our lives.
- **HUMOR**: We joke about unwanted experiences instead of feeling them and taking them seriously.

When we improve our capacity to hold the emotional alarms that arise when we're hurt—or hurting others—we don't need to be so afraid of our histories and mistakes, or to devalue the people who bring them to our awareness. We can teach our youth to be strong enough to learn about difficult topics such as systemic inequities, the climate crisis, and the dark parts of our national histories (like genocides, slavery, and colonization) without worrying that they can't handle the discomfort of the truth. We don't need to candy-coat our pasts to create fake patriotism. We can teach them that pride comes from the hard work of building a collective that we can be proud of, not from believing propaganda that we're better than everyone else without any effort. Only by sharing with them all the times our ancestors have harmed, been harmed, and healed can they learn from these experience so they don't have to repeat our mistakes.

WHEN THE PAST HASN'T PASSED

Our pasts can also imprison us to repeatedly relive the feelings of traumatic memories, as Toni Morrison's novel *Beloved* illustrates, with her protagonist's many flashbacks of the horrific abuse and loss she experienced as a slave at Sweet Home plantation nearly two decades before:

> Unfortunately, her brain was devious. She might be hurrying across a field, running practically, to get to the pump quickly and rinse the chamomile sap from her legs. Nothing else would be in her mind . . . Then something. The splash of water, the sight of her shoes and stockings awry on the path where she had flung them; or Here Boy lapping in the puddle near her feet, and suddenly there was Sweet Home rolling, rolling, rolling out before her eyes, and although there was not a leaf on that farm that did not make her want to scream, it rolled itself out before her in shameless beauty.

When memories of the past dominate our attention like this, we can use the same strategy of anchoring ourselves in the present by shifting our attention to the sensations visiting our body right now. We can integrate and process these past thoughts within the present feelings in the body, returning our system back into balance, where the past is no longer split off and dominating our awareness.

If inhabiting our body sensations pushes us outside our window of tolerance, again, we first work to regulate through the skills of the last chapter. With practice, we become more able to move our attention to wherever it's most helpful. We can begin by bringing our attention to our external senses—the sights, smells, and sounds around us—as they tend to be experienced more neutrally. Then we can slowly work our way toward bringing awareness to our more neutral body sensations, perhaps the earlobe, elbows, or feet. Finally, we can move our attention toward the edges, and then the center, of our more heated body sensations.

If this is too intense, we can move our attention between a neutral focus in the body or environment and then back to the edges of the more heated body sensations like a pendulum, practicing spending a little more time in the intense sensations and then taking respite again in a neutral spot, and back again. If you struggle to practice this approach without overactivating or deactivating, especially when trauma is pulling you into the past, you may find it helpful to begin practicing with someone skilled in co-regulation to support you in the process, such as a therapist.

NOTICING OUR EMOTIONAL SIGNATURES

Learning how to hold emotions in our bodies gives us power. If we build the strength to notice and comfortably feel all the emotional alarms that come along with living a full and meaningful life, then even the arrival of unpleasant emotions can be used to help us move toward our goals, instead of their ugly cloaks scaring us to run in the opposite direction.

Each unique emotion passes through us in predictable yet individual ways. We can learn to recognize the nuances of different emotional signals when they arise in a new moment and identify situations that typically induce these reactions in us. Rather than fusing with these states, thinking *I'm angry*, for example, we can depersonalize the alarm and remind ourselves of its impermanence by observing, *An anger alarm is passing through me right now*. Simply labeling emotions can help us regulate them. When we identify emotional states with words, we dampen the intensity of the emotion by bringing our prefrontal cortex back online.

You can practice observing and labeling the components of each emotional signature for a variety of emotional alarms, noticing when these alarms arise and recording how it feels in your body.

FOR EACH EMOTION LISTED BELOW, ANSWER THE FOLLOWING QUESTIONS:

- What types of situations typically induce this signal?
- Body Sensations: What do you feel in your body as you scan the different parts?
  - What's the temperature of different areas?
  - What areas feel more tight or more loose?
  - What areas feel more heavy or more light?
  - Is there any movement in any areas (such as shaking, pulsing, tingling)?

Joy

_____

Anger

_____

Fear

_____

Sadness

_____

Guilt

_____

Shame

_____

There are many other emotions that you can explore in the same way. Try observing your signatures for other emotional signals you typically encounter, such as jealousy, envy, love, or disgust.

THE MIXED-UP MESSAGES OF SECONDARY EMOTIONS

You'll probably notice that you are more comfortable experiencing some emotions, while you're more likely to avoid or defend against others. We might develop patterns of preferring certain emotions over others, switching the primary emotion that is giving us important information about our current experience into secondary ones that feel more comfortable. Our emotional habits are shaped by what was modeled to us in our families, communities, and cultures, and what we've learned is safe to express within these contexts.

For example, perhaps expressions of the more vulnerable emotions such as sadness, fear, guilt, or shame were not safe in our social worlds, so we were taught to switch them to the more powerful emotion of anger as a secondary emotion instead. Or perhaps anger felt scary growing up, because it was unsafe in our environments to stand up for ourselves, so we've learned to switch appropriate anger into secondary fear, shame, or guilt. Sometimes, any expression of emotion feels unsafe, so we react to all our emotions with secondary shame or we shut down for having them. In this way, we develop habitual emotional reactions to our emotions themselves.

When we've learned that the primary emotion is undesirable or unsafe, we switch it to another emotion. As I've struggled with a sensitive nervous system and anxiety all my life, when I experience fear, I often have a secondary emotion of shame for feeling so much fear. This happens a lot when I'm public speaking. When I notice the valid fear come up, because everybody is staring at me and that's a pretty weird experience, I then feel more fear for having such visible fear, making me more physically anxious. I also feel secondary shame, with old familiar stories that others will judge or reject me for appearing anxious. Social anxiety is often a combination of the fear-of-fear cycle and this secondary shame for feeling fear.

The challenge with secondary emotions is that the primary emotion's message and appropriate actions get lost in translation. We now hear the louder message of the secondary emotion and use its signals to guide us, missing the important information and appropriate actions that go with the primary emotion's read of the actual situation in front of us. It's like we've asked our GPS for directions to the local strip mall to take our kids to the toy shop, but it leads us to a strip club instead.

We often make the switch into secondary emotions without even being aware of it or noticing the primary emotion underneath. For example, if it has never been safe to admit mistakes, when we're called in for making a harmful comment, we might not feel safe to feel the guilt that would push us to be accountable and improve our behavior. Instead, we slip unconsciously into the fight-or-flight of anger or shame, blaming the person we've harmed for how we feel, or avoiding them at all costs. Learning to build more comfort within a larger window of tolerance for our emotions can allow us to be much more skillful and intentional in our actions.

We can more explicitly practice allowing and acceptance skills when working to build comfort with all our internal experiences—even the ones we've been conditioned to see as ugly—with an exercise called R.A.I.N., first developed twenty years ago by Vipassana meditation teacher Michele McDonald. R.A.I.N. outlines the steps we can practice when bringing kind awareness to challenging experiences. The *N* in McDonald's original exercise stood for *nonidentification*, reminding us that each passing experience is not personal. Because the research for self-compassion has grown since the practice was first conceived, many teachers have changed the *N* to stand for *nurture*, to explicitly remind us of the impact of relating to each experience with self-compassion and tenderness. We can try to approach every step of R.A.I.N. with nonidentification, and all three of the insights we observe with extended mindfulness practice, what Ruth King summarizes as life not being personal, permanent, or perfect.

R.A.I.N. EXERCISE

1. RECOGNIZE:
   - Where are you on the dial of activation?
   - What body sensations, feelings, thoughts, and action urges do you notice?
   - What reactions to these experiences are present?

2. ALLOW:
   - Try to relate to your internal experiences without judgment or need for them to be any different than they already are. Perhaps saying to yourself, *It's already here. May it be just as it is. It's okay. It's safe to feel this. I consent to these inner experiences being here.* Or simply add a *Yes* to whatever arises.

3. INVESTIGATE THE BODY SENSATIONS:
   - Move out of your head and into your body: What body sensations are arising right now? Scan the body to observe the unique dance of the spectrum of different temperatures, levels of tension and heaviness, and changing movements in each part.

4. NURTURE:
   - Ask yourself how to best care for these inner experiences. What do they need? Do they need validation? What's the most compassionate way to meet this experience? What important information are they offering you that can help you care for yourself and others?

WORKING WITH PHYSICAL PAIN AND SYMPTOMS

"My chest hurts," my son told me one morning. After training as a medical doctor, anyone who says the magic phrase *chest pain* gets immediately triaged to the front of my attention and care. Jumping up, I quickly listed off all the questions on the chest pain algorithm.

As I examined his body with precision, he told me, "I think it's because it's Remembrance Day today," breaking me out of my doctor trance.

"That makes so much sense, love. What does it bring up for you?" I responded, finally attuning to what he needed in the moment. We chatted about how sad and scary war is, especially in the context of the violence around the world right now. He told me how he noticed anxiety in his body come up as chest pain when he thought about it. We continued to validate his feelings and normalize how our emotions and thoughts talk to us through our bodies in pain or noisy physical symptoms.

I laughed to myself after, realizing that my young son seemed more able to link his emotions with body symptoms than I could as a psychotherapist. I had quickly let my old autopilot of medical doctor mode dominate that moment of his distress, forgetting that our physical and emotional symptoms are intertwined within the same neural pathways. Emotional threats are physically painful and physical threats are emotionally painful. They're entangled in a shared network.

The separation of mental and physical health only lasted for a quick bender in Western history, but its hangover continues to impact medicine to this day. It began with philosopher René Descartes proposing the dualism between mind and body in the seventeenth century. Western doctors jumped at the opportunity to divorce the body from the mind, since the dominant orthodox Christian views of a united body and soul prohibited the dissection of human anatomy to ensure the soul would ascend to heaven.[7] By separating the two, the body could be studied, birthing the biomedical model that reduced humans to the study of our measurable, isolated parts—from our bio-chemistry to physiology and anatomy.[8]

We soon returned to our holistic views of the interconnected body and mind, with physicians now learning the bio-psycho-social-spiritual model of health. But the intergenerational learning of the dualistic biomedical model from our past resurfaces in both physicians and patients alike, in the same way that I carry my ancestors' wisdom, traumas, and tendency to tap dance in the kitchen, just like my long-deceased grandmother.

If we've been raised in families, cultures, or health-care systems where mental health symptoms are stigmatized or minimized while physical health complaints are respected and offered treatment, we might notice that our emotional distress is unconsciously conditioned to come out only in physical ways, such as gastrointestinal problems, dizziness, fatigue, chronic pain, or any other symptoms that we might label as somatization—the expression of emotional symptoms through the body.

In cultures that don't share in these old misconceptions of mind-body separation, such as in holistic Chinese cultural traditions, one's physical, mental, spiritual, and social health symptoms are not seen as seperate. For example, during the Cultural Revolution, many of the large numbers of Chinese citizens targeted by the political opposition became sick with *shenjing shuairuo*, a condition characterized by the entangled psychological and physical symptoms of insomnia, fatigue, and headaches.[9]

Because physical stress can lead to both physical and emotional symptoms and emotional stress can lead to emotional and physical symptoms, we can use the same strategies to manage both emotional and physical pain and distress in our bodies. The first step, as always, is to pay attention to what message the alarm is signaling. If we have a new physical symptom, such as pain or fatigue, we want to investigate what threat it's trying to communicate. Sometimes, pain or physical symptoms are telling us to rest the area or set a healthy boundary in our lives. Sometimes the symptom gets louder to alert us to see a professional for diagnosis and treatment or to change our behaviors. These are helpful alarms.

But our bodies also give us false alarms. We might get stuck in chronic pain cycles or physical symptoms that have been worked up by health-care providers and don't indicate an acute problem we can fix. In these cases, we can learn to surf the pain and physical discomfort using the same strategies that we just learned to manage emotional pain. We can move our attention away from the unhelpful cloak of thoughts and reactions about the discomfort that only makes it worse. We can then shift it toward noticing the physical body sensations themselves, observing their temperature, heaviness, tension, and movement, or practice R.A.I.N., just as we did with emotional pain. We can also notice when our attention is being dominated by thoughts about the symptoms, or tunnel-visioning into one area of the body, and broaden our spotlight of awareness so that all our senses are in balance by exploring sensations in other areas of the body or our connection to others and our environment.

BRINGING OURSELVES INTO BALANCE

We heal by bringing all the parts of our mind-body-social-spiritual system—and the world around us—back into balance, rather than being dominated by any one part. When we're able to access our different states of activation in all of the nuanced emotional flavors they come in, we're granted the flexibility to employ whatever strategy best matches each new situation. We gain more power to respond in helpful ways when we're no longer stuck reacting in only one rigid pattern that dominates all the other more skillful responses to that specific moment.

For example, sometimes, we react to every stressful situation with our fight mode of anger and blame. While we learned the emotional pattern years ago to match a situation or culture that it served at that time, it likely doesn't match the specific needs of the wide variety of moments we face every day that require more flexible and unique responses. We may have been conditioned to believe that anger is the only safe or helpful emotion based on our past environments and relationships. But as we gain more comfort in feeling all our emotions, we get to add these additional alarms to our toolbox.

Similarly, if we've learned, like I have, to habitually deactivate into overthinking, distraction, or denial instead of feeling our alarms in the body whenever a stress arises, we miss out on all the important emotional information and can't use it to attune to others or act in ways that match the situation's needs. By building a wider window of tolerance in holding our emotions, we don't need to run away so much, losing their valuable functions.

When emotional wounds carry intense pain or shame, we tend to disown them, compartmentalizing and splitting them off from the rest of our consciousness, until we're pushed into fully inhabiting them with the right trigger. When we're fragmented in this way, with our different parts not integrated and aware of each other, it can feel jarring and confusing as we suddenly inhabit a separate state of mind and body, as if we're suddenly possessed by a foreign entity. As we lose access to the other parts of our system in these split-off states, we no longer have the capacity to even see what triggered it, leaving us powerless and feeling as though this distressing state came "out of the blue." As a result, our attempts to protect ourselves from the painful emotional state by splitting it off makes us more distressed, as we experience the emotion and its associated body sensations, thoughts, and urges in an all-or-nothing way.

When we build more comfort and acceptance in painful feelings, we don't need to split them off. We can keep them integrated and connected to the rest of our consciousness so that when they arise, we still have our other parts available to help us understand what's happening and cope with it.

When I'm activated into a shame wave, suddenly believing I'm an imposter or that everyone hates me, instead of believing that I'm now a pariah and should quit or hide before I get rejected, I can notice these shame-related emotions and thoughts and acknowledge I'm temporarily hijacked by shame. Then I can ground myself in the present by feeling the sensations of this reaction in my body and use this alarm to be curious if I'm in a rejecting or psychologically unsafe environment right now. If not, I can acknowledge that it's a false alarm from old wounds arising, and offer myself compassion for having to experience these so often, just as I'd run myself a hot bath if my back hurt.

When a protective alarm sounds, we can both feel it in the body *and* observe it while it's happening (or soon after), as if we have one foot in the experience of feeling the alarm and one grounded in the observing stance of stability—the mountain noticing the intricate dance of the storm. If we don't fear, judge, or get stuck fully identifying with the passing storm that arises, we can clearly see and ride the sensations of its protective message without getting lost in the fog.

We've explored already how our early attachment to caregivers helps us learn to regulate our emotions through co-regulation. When our caregivers haven't had the capacity to help us co-regulate, we might struggle to bring our emotional responses into conscious awareness on our own. Instead, when our alarms sound, it may feel like mysterious forces are controlling how we behave and feel, because we can't identify or make sense of all the parts making up the storm.

Even if we haven't had the opportunity to learn these skills in childhood, it's never too late to learn to bring our emotional reactions into awareness and make sense of all their moving parts. Sometimes, we need the help of a professional to get us started. Therapists can help us find the sweet spot of inviting in just enough discomfort to gradually regain a fuller range of emotions without pushing us too much into intolerable distress.

THE OVERMONITORING OF ANXIETY

With repeated exposure to a wide range of emotional activation in a safe setting, we can extinguish the implicit learning attached to emotions that mistakenly fused the feelings of the alarms themselves with the dangerous situations they're signaling. For example, many people with anxiety get stuck in a fear-of-fear cycle, where the body sensations and feelings of the alarms themselves are believed to be dangerous instead of the perceived threat that these alarms are signaling. Fear pushes us to be hypervigilant. But while scanning our environments for threats in hostile environments is helpful, overmonitoring our body sensations when scared only makes our anxiety worse. For years, I struggled with this kind of anxiety, excessively scanning my body for any changes in sensations that might indicate a future panic attack or disease. Then, when I'd inevitably find something noisy in my body—my heart racing or my breath feeling tight—my alarm system would be triggered again by the body sensations of its own alarm, spiraling me into a full-blown panic attack in an instant.

As we learned in Chapter Two, in systems theory, we call this a positive feedback loop. Most of the time, our systems communicate and right themselves back into balance with negative feedback loops. For example, our anger alarm rings when there's an intrusion on our boundaries, so it helps us assert these boundaries to bring the system back into balance, quieting the alarm. But the fear-of-fear cycle switches us into the opposite response where our alarms create more alarms, pushing us further out of balance.

When we notice we're conditioned into this cycle, we can break it by building comfort with our emotional alarms by exposing ourselves to them in safe settings, such as with a therapist or in a quiet room, and anchor ourselves in the present by focusing on the body sensations themselves rather than the scary stories we've created about them. With practice, we realize it's okay to have noisy bodies and no longer misinterpret the alarm itself as dangerous. We can retrain ourselves to observe, experience, and interpret the body sensations of the alarms as safe and helpful, while moving our awareness to evaluate the situation that the alarm is trying to alert us to. It works: I haven't had a panic attack in decades.

This exposure approach can also desensitize the intensity of alarms conditioned to past or misperceived dangers that we no longer need in our current environment. When exposure therapy was first conceptualized, we'd focus on the external trigger—driving after a car accident, going to a party or grocery store—and expose ourselves to the situation that we'd implicitly associated with the threat again and again. We still do this, but it's less accessible because most people who are afraid of flying or the dentist don't get enough exposure to these situations to decondition their anxiety response, nor is it easy to bring a therapist along for the ride.

Luckily, we can simply expose ourselves to the emotions and body sensations themselves within a safe setting to desensitize unhelpful alarms.[10] We can bring to mind threatening situations or induce the noisy physical sensations of the alarms by hyperventilating, spinning in a chair, breathing through a straw, or exercising to bring on physical activation. Then, we can practice surfing the sensations of the feelings in our bodies to update our interpretation of the experience as safe, diminishing the alarm's intensity. In this way, we build comfort with the noisy body sensations, thoughts, and feelings of the anxiety response. We learn to see these responses as imperfect, impersonal, and impermanent storms passing through our awareness.

It's important to remember that simply reexperiencing the threatening situation or emotion isn't enough to desensitize our alarms. We must do so in a safer context than before, either in a more secure environment or relationship, or with healthier skills to manage it. Otherwise, we risk strengthening our threat response by continuing to feel overwhelmed and unable to cope with the situation.

For example, if we end up stuck in our heads ruminating about negative experiences without coupling those thoughts with a new sense of safety or capacity to handle them, we amplify these distressing thoughts and feelings in a vicious cycle that worsens our suffering. This can happen with panic attacks or PTSD flashbacks when we feel repeatedly overwhelmed by intrusive anxiety without having the skills or support to manage the distress, so it continues to feel unsafe despite numerous exposures.

In CBT, we illustrate the intensity of anxiety with the anxiety equation: anxiety = estimation of danger/estimation of ability to cope with it.

Even though we have so little control over the threats in our outer worlds, we can work to build our capacity to cope with these threats when they inevitably occur. Exposure therapy helps us develop the confidence that we can handle the distressing event and its associated feelings and still be okay.

Neuroscientists are now discovering that our memories aren't permanent or perfect representations of the past, because they undergo multiple revisions and additions as we recollect and update them to adapt to new contexts. We can update our memory and its associated emotions by coupling it with new emotional experiences in its present context, softening its edges for the next time it gets triggered.[11]

Our primary subcortical emotional systems can also regulate our learning and information processing from the bottom up. If we couple the emotional activation of past memories with our ABCs of regulation (agency, bonding, containment) or play, care, lust, and seeking, we can update them in less distressing forms.[12] For example, if we choose to return to the location of an old wound with a friend, we update the emotional memory evoked from the activating situation with the care of our friend, the agency of choosing to go there with new skills to practice, and perhaps even a playful approach to the challenge. Or if we have a therapist evoke an old trauma memory in session, we can soften the memory by adding in the agency of practicing kind attention to our body sensations and the care of co-regulation with the safety of the therapist. If we bring up a past event that arose in the context of needing to fawn in fear or shame while inhibiting anger to keep us safe at that time, we can introduce the agency of experiencing and validating the anger that matches the situation's unmet need, injustice, or violation, which we now are safe to express.[13] Even practicing our own kind attention adds this same agency and care.

Researchers keep finding that psychotherapy, regardless of the style of therapy offered, is most effective and satisfying when deep emotions are experienced in session, arguing that emotional experiencing may be the common pathway to therapeutic change.[14] Psychotherapy outcomes improve even more when we also learn to listen to the messages of our emotional alarms to make meaning and solve problems.[15] While it's uncomfortable, psychotherapy that reactivates our emotions creates longer-lasting benefits than approaches that only focus on building insight and rational thinking.[16]

FEELING OURSELVES TO HEAL OUR WORLD

In *What It Takes to Heal*, Prentis Hemphill describes working as a therapist the day they learned of seventeen-year-old Trayvon Martin's murder, in yet another act of anti-Black racism, as he walked home from buying a bag of Skittles and a watermelon drink at his neighborhood store. "It was all I could do to maintain my composure, to act like a 'therapist' and resist pushing open every door and bringing us all together to cry it out in the hallways," they wrote. "There was something disingenuous about trying to fit each client's emotions neatly into personal therapeutic rooms when what they were feeling was never only individual."

When Martin's killer was acquitted, Hemphill went straight from their clinic to the streets, as the city erupted in protests, which they described as "electric, one of those rare moments in life when you can feel the raw power that exists when people come together . . . We were restoring our sense of power that is lost in violation. It was its own kind of healing. As much as I wanted individual therapy for every one of my clients, I wanted them to have this feeling too."

Hemphill felt how connected they all were in sharing their grief, not only for Martin, but for all the ghosts of each other's pasts. "I walked among people I didn't know and yet knew deeply," they wrote. "It's not practical to imagine that we can feel the weight of historical trauma as one person. This is why we meet in the streets. As much as mass protests and direct action are about putting strategic pressure on opposition, they are often a gathering space for our grief and pain because they are too big to feel alone . . . A community, a society, becomes one, remains one, I think, through shared feeling."

When we disconnect from our feelings, we also disconnect from our belonging to others and the web of life around us. Focusing on our feelings isn't a luxury, self-centered, or frivolous. It's how we open up to heal ourselves, each other, and the world that's making us sick. Whether we unite in protest, purpose, ceremony, worship, music, dance, sport, or any of the other beautifully diverse ways we join in community, we strengthen our connection through feeling together. And through feeling together, we strengthen our capacity to hold the pain.

Imagine how brave we can be when we build the strength to feel all the emotions that arise as we face the world? How would you choose to live if you weren't afraid to feel?

EIGHT

DON'T BELIEVE EVERYTHING YOU THINK

We do not see things as they are, we see them as we are.

—ANAÏS NIN

———————

"WHAT'S NATURE SCHOOL?" A GROWN-UP ASKED ONE OF MY SON'S PRESCHOOL CLASS-mates.

"Nature means being naked," she answered with confidence.

Let's leave aside the discussion of why so many psychiatrists choose to send their kids to roll around in a giant mud pit instead of learning any formal academics in their early years and examine this girl's answer.

The world is an uncertain place, only providing us with small pieces of information. This girl goes to "nature school." At nature school, the kids often get so dirty playing outside that they strip off their muddy clothes before changing into clean ones. Therefore, she makes associations and inferences to fill in the gaps of uncertainty. *Nature* must mean being naked.

Our brains do this all the time. We're so uncomfortable with the threat of uncertainty that the moment we have gaps in a story about our experiences, we fill them in with our best assumptions, which turns our thoughts into fiction. Our brains jump to assumptions and make rules and frameworks for how the world works with implicit learning, without us even being aware of these puppet masters working behind the scenes. It happens so fast that we don't realize that the resulting thoughts it creates are just thoughts and not accurate reflections of reality.

Thoughts are stories that our brains come up with to help us survive in our dangerous and unpredictable worlds. Our brains recognize patterns in our past to best predict the rewards and threats of our present and future. A predictable environment is a safe one: we need to know that the fish bite every dawn and the cougars come out at dusk. Life feels coherent when we have a sense of control and certainty over it. Otherwise, we become very anxious.

Our brains even reward us with dopamine when we recognize and complete patterns. When we fill in the gaps of an ambiguous experience in our environment with a more certain thought, we get a very reinforcing dopamine hit, even if the thought is incorrect. For this reason, therapists often refer to thoughts as "the story I'm telling myself." Because our negativity bias helps us survive, catastrophizing with worst-case scenarios—it's better to be safe than sorry, after all—we often fill in the gaps with themes of danger and rejection. Our brains would rather make up a miserable story than face an uncertain one.

Imagine you're meeting a friend and they haven't shown up. You check your phone and message them, and still no answer. We can first practice making our implicit reactions explicit by bringing awareness to all the different parts of our inner experience:

- WHAT body sensations do you notice (temperature, heaviness, tension, movement)?
- WHERE are you on the dial of activation?
- ARE you aware of a specific emotion present?
- WHAT actions do you feel urged to take?
- WHAT story are you telling yourself about what just happened?

I've offered this exercise with countless participants to demonstrate that we all come up with different stories about the exact same fact: the friend didn't show up. The key to the exercise is that it's missing information, just like most of our real-life experiences. Because our minds can't stand uncertainty, we fill in the gaps with fiction, without being aware that we're doing it. But these stories then affect how we feel and act.

Some people assume that something bad happened to their friend and feel fear, wanting to take actions to ensure they're okay. Others believe their friend is acting like a jerk who doesn't value their time, feeling anger and the desire to shoot off a heated text. Some think their friend doesn't like them, feeling sadness or shame and the urge to withdraw or hide from the situation. Still others worry they've made a mistake or offended the friend, feeling guilt and a need to check in and repair the relationship. The list could go on with all the ways we fill in the gaps to write a creative work of fiction.

How we feel and act is a consequence not only of the situation we find ourselves in, but how we interpret it. Unfortunately, our interpretations are often inaccurate and overly pessimistic. These automatic thoughts usually pop up outside of our awareness, so we end up distressed or demoralized and don't even know why.

Thinking is an imprecise process, what cognitive psychologists call "a kernel of truth, surrounded by a shell of inference."[1] In addition to our need for certainty and that helpful yet painful negativity bias we use to survive, thoughts are also influenced by our collective culture, intergenerational learning, personal history, safety of the present environment, current emotional state, and our behaviors.

I wonder if the story you created about your friend not showing up feels familiar. Cognitive therapists talk of our "top ten hits" to show that we often play variants of the same thoughts over and over, regardless of the situation we find ourselves in. In this way, our storytelling stays on the same theme based on our implicit rules and patterns that we've learned in life—the *others can't be trusted, I'm not enough,* or *one false step and I'm rejected* tracks. These stories reflect the personal, collective, and intergenerational learning we accumulate to keep us away from harm.

When we or our ancestors have been exposed to more dangers, then our stories will carry louder warnings. We may have more false alarms because we've adapted to meet the increased risk of our environments, or that of our ancestors. For this reason, I'm careful to stay away from calling our resulting thoughts "distorted." Yes, they are often false alarms for the present situation, biased toward themes of danger and rejection. But they come from somewhere valid—either we or our ancestors have learned that these warning signals are essential to survival. It's a healthy adaptation, especially when you're able to identify what's a false alarm from past learning and what's an accurate assessment of the threat of the present situation. We want our fire alarm to go off every time there's smoke. But we also need to look around to see if there are really flames in front of us, or if it's just our bagel burning in the toaster.

The present environment also affects the stories we tell. If we were meeting up at our favorite place, where everyone feels friendly and safe, our stories might be softer than if we showed up at an uninviting event or new community where we really needed that friend to help us feel comfortable.

Our behaviors also affect our stories. If we hadn't left our home for a while, and this was the first time we attempted to socialize, we might have a very different story than if we meet up with others all the time and have received a lot of positive feedback from these encounters to disprove our more cynical stories. (We will explore how our behaviors affect our mental health in Chapter Nine.)

Finally, our current emotions and level of activation affect our stories—a lot. What if we just got dumped, lost our job or housing, or faced an act of discrimination or injustice, and then we arrived to meet our friend and they didn't show up? The feeling of anger, fear, sadness, or shame we arrived with will flavor the stories we create in this new situation. If we just felt invisible and devalued at a meeting, then the story we create about our friend's absence will likely include these themes. But if we just came from an empowering protest, a heart-to-heart with someone who values us, or an event where we felt that we belonged and mattered, and then arrived to find no friend, we might interpret the situation as much less threatening. Same situation, different story. Cognitive therapists describe this phenomenon as "feelings giving birth to thoughts."[2]

Let's flesh out an example of how all these factors interact to create a complicated mess of creative fiction. I really struggled in medical school. It wasn't studying for the exams that stressed me out; it was the threat of making mistakes and harming real people that kept me sweating right through my white coat. My body still tenses at the beep of a pager, and there's a certain scent of generic laundry detergent that brings me right back to the sleepless nights of our call shifts at the hospital, when I would check, and then recheck, potassium levels, vitals, urine output, even that damn pager to ensure I didn't miss something that would cause harm.

I was painfully anxious all the time, obsessed with thoughts that I would harm someone and that others would realize I was an imposter—that I didn't belong. These two stories were my top tracks. Most people assume that anxiety is synonymous with fear. But anxiety itself is not a specific emotion. It's a broad term that describes a dark cloud of discomfort, experienced in both our bodies and brains. While anxiety is often linked to fear, it can also relate to stories of causing harm—that is, guilt—or of a part of us being rejected—as with shame.

It's not themes of fear that drive my anxiety. When people see me hanging off cliffs or hucking myself down mountains on my bike, they assume I couldn't possibly be the anxious type. But guilt and shame are my game. So, why was I primed to have so many anxious thoughts during medical school?

THOUGHTS ARE CONTAGIOUS

Thoughts that lead to guilt and shame are contagious, collectively shared among a culture. People joke about their "Catholic guilt," but they are talking about an important phenomenon of how our inner psychologies are socially transmitted in groups. We internalize stories of guilt, shame, anger, or any emotion from the cultures that raise us.

Most of our social learning is helpful: we learn languages, ethics, and healthy ways to connect with friends, colleagues, and lovers through internalizing the beliefs and behaviors of others. Sometimes, though, we sacrifice our individual freedoms and needs to maintain the cohesion and social order of the group, especially in cultures that are less tolerant of diversity. This may work on average for the dominant members of the group, but it can harm those who don't fit the narrow criteria to belong. Whether it's social systems that exclude or subordinate groups of people, specific interpretations of religious scriptures that shun diversity, or groups passing on shame-based learning from the generations before them because "that's the way it's always been," social learning can evolve too slowly to help us thrive in the new environments we find ourselves in. These thoughts habitually pop into our mind on autopilot, as automatic thoughts outside of our awareness. But as we discussed already, autopilot is the past's solution to today's problem.

When we're socialized within cultures that uphold the dynamics of domination, division, and dehumanization, no one wins. Raised as a white middle-class settler in a country built on inequities, racism, and colonization, I could always sense the privileges I held at the expense of others, leaving me marinating in guilt and shame much of the time.

At the same time, while this unearned power and privilege makes my queerness quite safe in the communities I now inhabit, as a kid and teen of the 1980s and '90s, there wasn't much representation of queer life in my world, leaving me with a vague, yet profound, sense of not belonging if I were to show my true self. We were the generation when most of us came out after high school, when we felt safe enough to do so.

I wasn't raised conservative, nor was I involved in any form of organized religion. Instead, I grew up learning about progressive politics at the dinner table in a diverse area of Vancouver. Neither my family nor my friends were overtly homophobic. But we're always marinating in the subtle messages of our wider culture that constantly monitors and advises us on how we show up in the world. Stories of guilt and shame, internalized from my society, quietly nudged me into conceal-ment, without my even being aware of it.

Upon graduation, I spent much of my early adulthood in coun-tries where same-sex relationships were illegal or rejected. Already socially anxious, people-pleasing, and surrounded by a heteronorma-tive culture both at home and abroad, I concealed this part of myself that didn't fit the society around me. I only felt safe to be openly queer when my collective culture became more inclusive, with greater rep-resentation and acceptance of the beautiful spectrum of gender and sexual expression. And only when I shared these parts of myself with those who were safe to hold them did I feel real belonging, healing the stories of shame and guilt that I carried for so many years.

What messages have you internalized from your culture? What does it mean when most photos in children's books, magazines, and textbooks show people of the dominant culture? Or that our justice system disproportionally polices, convicts, and kills specific groups? Or that the media links beauty and health with body shapes, and masculin-ity with dominance and an absence of emotions? We are constantly—and often subtly—taking in stories of worth, belonging, and thus guilt and shame when we don't fit those narrow definitions of the dominant culture of what it takes to be (shame) or do (guilt) to belong.

HOW THE PAST HAS NOT PASSED

Our individual learning from our close relationships, too, especially from our family of origin and early attachment to caregivers, influ-ences our thoughts. One of my attachment figures had to hold a lot of anxiety in their life. And when it overwhelmed them, they numbed the distress with alcohol, like so many do. This culturally learned pattern of coping with uncomfortable emotions with substances led to an addiction that I interpreted, from my child's mind, as all my fault.

In situations when we're forced to face our utter powerlessness in the world, we often create the fantasy that it's our fault, to reclaim our power. *Aha! I've figured out why my caregiver, whom I depend on and love more than anything in the world, is unavailable. The whole world's not out of order; it's just me who's bad. If only I was good enough, then they would choose me over alcohol, then the world wouldn't feel so bad. I just need to figure out how to be better, then everything will be okay.*

But I never could. I tried adopting perfectionism, people-pleasing, caregiving, and charisma, but nothing I did seemed to work. My childlike thinking split the world into all good or bad; I didn't see the complex gray of reality. This paired with my genetic wiring, which had adapted to meet the dangers faced by my ancestors, led to symptoms of obsessive-compulsive disorder (OCD), a condition of thinking-dominance fixated on stories of guilt and shame, in an elusive battle to think away and undo the perceived bad within me.

As my caregiver continued to conceal their addiction in shame, quietly relapsing behind closed doors and going away for numerous stints in rehab, I too inherited this shame, hiding the disorder of our family. It makes sense, then, that I've continued this pattern of thinking that attributes everything, even things outside of my control, as my fault. Like so many, I fell into these omnipotent—albeit distressing— stories instead of accepting my powerlessness, at least until therapy helped me see this pattern of thinking so I can identify when I project it onto new experiences.

Our stories and adaptations, especially to potentially dangerous environments, can also be passed on through the generations. As I mentioned before, I was raised by my grandmother, whose parents and siblings fled Russia after the failed Russian Revolution of 1905, when the Tsar's regime violently retaliated against Jews, Poles, and Ukrainians, because many of them fought with the diverse alliance of workers, peasants, and the military to revolt against systemic discrimination.

Her parents changed their name when they settled in North America, still afraid that being different would be a death sentence. I notice how the inner dialogue I carry about myself—that it's dangerous to be different—follows the same theme that my family carried from generations ago.

SHAME THRIVES IN PSYCHOLOGICALLY UNSAFE SETTINGS

When I arrived on the hospital wards as a medical student and then resident, I was already conditioned by the negativity bias, the collective culture around me, and my personal history to interpret the world through my hypersensitized shame and guilt alarms. Then, when my new environment adopted the practice of shame-based learning, in a profession fueled by the high-stakes consequences of harm and perfectionism, the threat of making a mistake activated these beliefs even more: *I'm an imposter here and don't belong* and *I'm going to cause harm.*

Epidemics of guilt and shame spread quickly in social environments that lack psychological safety. In his book *The 4 Stages of Psychological Safety,* Timothy Clark defines psychological safety as needing both respect and permission to have autonomy within a group. He describes four stages of psychological safety: (1) Inclusion Safety, the permission to interact with others as a human being and belong to a group; (2) Learner Safety, the permission to learn and make mistakes without criticism; (3) Contributor Safety, the permission to work independently and contribute new ideas; and (4) Challenger Safety, the permission to challenge the status quo in good faith and respectfully disagree.

When I teach workshops about vulnerability in medicine to students and physicians, they immediately explain that their environments aren't psychologically safe enough to enjoy the benefits of practicing vulnerability. They're right. Vulnerability is a privilege, only available and helpful to those of us whose social settings are safe enough to take off our armor without injury. It would be emotionally harmful to teach my students to strip off their defenses when they could be shamed and guilted in an environment that isn't psychologically safe. That's why I also teach leaders, mentors, and supervisors themselves, those who have the power to change the psychological safety of our culture.

FEELINGS GIVE BIRTH TO THOUGHTS

When we arrive in a new situation already feeling an emotion, such as my familiar state of guilt and shame that I frequently find myself in, then these emotions dictate how we write new stories about our experiences. This is particularly powerful when we live with depression or anxiety. If we are experiencing a depressive episode, we are stuck in feelings of sadness, anger, guilt, or shame. These chronic feelings color all our new experiences to create a pessimistic running commentary on our day-to-day life. Because so many of our thoughts arise implicitly, we find ourselves marinating in dark thoughts that perpetuate our depression without being aware of it.

When I facilitate groups for people living with depression, I have participants fill out the Depressive Automatic Thoughts Questionnaire. I ask them how true these thoughts are when they are most and least depressed. The thoughts listed on the questionnaire reflect the top ten tracks for people living with depression: *I've let people down, I'm worthless, I'm a failure, My life's a mess, I feel so helpless, My future is bleak,* and so on. To those participants in my groups experiencing anxiety symptoms, I offer similar questionnaires that reflect common anxious thoughts: *If someone is late, I assume there's an accident; If someone is hurt or offended by what I do, this means I am a bad person; People will think that there is something wrong with me if they see that I'm anxious; If I make a mistake, that means I am stupid;* and so on.

Participants are often surprised to see that everyone else in the group experiences similar thoughts. While depressed and anxious thoughts feel so personal and permanent, these stories are simply passing expressions of the mood states or feelings themselves. And sure enough, participants universally describe that when their depression and anxiety symptoms abate, the stories do, too. These thoughts don't disappear entirely but remain dormant and outside our awareness until the emotional state returns in a new storm.

When I work with people who struggle with episodic mood and anxiety disorders, I have them write down the stories they tell themselves about how they view themselves, the world, and others when they're experiencing few symptoms. Then when they relapse and these emotional storms bring with them their alarming stories, they can reference this list and be reminded of how just a few weeks or even days ago, they believed an entirely different narrative.

One of the great struggles we face in maintaining our mental health is emotion- and mood-dependent memory. When we are distressed or shut down, we don't have access to the stories we held when we were emotionally balanced. And when we're in balance, it's hard to imagine being distressed or shut down again. It's hard to have hope when we're marinating only in dark memories. In these moments, we need to trust that when our emotions and mood come back into balance, so will our thoughts. Sometimes, we need to borrow the hope of others and allow them keep us safe until our stories brighten up again.

In this way, we can see thoughts not as reflecting the truth of our situations, but as signals that give us information about our current mood or state of emotional activation. Just like a fever warns us that we may have an infection, pessimistic thoughts signal that we may be venturing into states of low mood, while self-doubting or unworthiness thoughts signal that we're activated into shame.

Yet we usually take our thoughts so personally. When they tell us we're a loser, it's hard to take a step back and see these familiar thought patterns as simply a symptom of the mood or emotional state that's visiting. When I start to notice old stories of not belonging or causing harm coming up, instead of automatically believing these thoughts, I can instead take an inventory of my life: Am I overstressed? Have I enough sleep, activity, social connection, and meaning in my life right now? Do I need to set healthier boundaries? Are there early steps I can take to catch these thought patterns before they cascade into a full-blown anxious or depressed state? It's just like when you notice a scratchy throat coming on and you decide to slow down and take care of yourself. It's easier to notice it early and be proactive than to try to pull ourselves out of a deep episode of depression or anxiety.

We also need to keep in mind how feelings give birth to thoughts when engaging in therapy, self-help, or other styles of healing work to process past trauma, loss, or relational challenges that occurred in specific emotional states of activation. If we only reflect on these experiences without feeling the emotional component in the body, we aren't gaining access to the actual stories, associations, and beliefs about ourselves, others, and the world that are fused with the experiences. Instead, we're thinking about that time from a different state of emotional activation, interpreting the situation from this entirely different lens that doesn't match what we thought in that moment. When this happens, the painful stories and beliefs remain split off and unprocessed until we're involuntarily triggered right back into them again, usually at the most inconvenient times.

NOTICING YOUR EMOTION-DEPENDENT THINKING

It can be helpful to observe our thoughts as we move through different emotional states throughout the week and document what stories about ourselves, others, and the world arise from these states.

FOR EACH EMOTION LISTED BELOW, ANSWER THE FOLLOWING QUESTIONS:

- What types of situations typically induce this signal?
- Body Sensations: What do you feel in your body as you scan the different parts?
  - What's the temperature of different areas?
  - What areas feel more tight or more loose?
  - What areas feel more heavy or more light?

> □ Is there any movement in any areas (such as shaking, pulsing, tingling)?
>
> □ What thoughts about yourself, others, and the world are present?

Joy

_____

Anger

_____

Fear

_____

Sadness

_____

Guilt

_____

Shame

_____

What do you notice when you compare your stories about yourself, others, and the world from different emotional states? We often are quite surprised to learn how widely our beliefs differ depending on our emotions and level of activation.

SEEING THOUGHTS JUST AS THOUGHTS

> Great doubt great enlightenment, little doubt little enlightenment, no doubt no enlightenment.
>
> —ZEN PROVERB

As someone who spent my early life plagued by painful and perpetual habits of thinking, I don't blame you if you wish we could learn ways to stop these pesky thoughts from ever arising. In fact, cognitive therapists have tried with "thought-stopping" practices. They would advise us to say or visualize some form of *Stop!* inside our mind when the challenging thought arose. As attractive and simple as it seems, this strategy actually backfires and makes the thoughts worse.[3] For example, try to not think about a turquoise banana for the next twenty seconds.

It's all you think about, right? The more we try to push these thoughts out of our heads, the more frequently and intensely they arise.

While postpartum depression is becoming well-known to the public, fewer people recognize postpartum anxiety, which is more common in new parents than depression.[4] When I lead postpartum mental health groups, I'm always struck that half of the participants describe OCD-like thinking (intrusive, repetitive, and unwanted thoughts that they can't get out of their heads) when sharing their anxious thoughts. Sometimes, they're recurrent obsessions about harm to their baby (like dropping them, cutting them with the knife they're using to prepare dinner, or rolling over on them in their sleep). After my first baby was born, I didn't sleep for months as I compulsively checked on him, plagued by terrifying and intrusive images of him stopping breathing. Other parents can't get intrusive and unwanted images of their baby's genitals out of their mind after changing a diaper. Because they then tell themselves the story that they must be bad for having these distressing images in their minds, the more they try to get them out of their head, the more intrusive and frequent the images become.

Studies show that parents with unwanted and intrusive OCD thoughts like these are the least likely of anyone to harm their babies.[5] In fact, we're predisposed to OCD from a strong genetic predisposition paired with high levels of conscientiousness and morality. (Of interest, OCD, attention-deficit hyperactivity disorder, and tic disorders are all highly genetically linked, what we call the *genetic triad*, and run strongly together in families.) Everyone sometimes gets odd, intrusive thoughts in their head of harm or any of the other things we may consider culturally undesirable to think. The difference is that people with OCD judge their thoughts as bad and try to stop them. This is why some religious teachings that judge our automatic thoughts (the ones that involuntarily pop into our heads) as sinful can amplify OCD symptoms. The more we try to push unwanted thoughts out of our head, the stronger they return.

When psychologists studied this, instructing participants to not think or feel something sad, they become more prone to anxious and depressive thoughts and symptoms.[6] While we can make our thoughts worse by trying to rid ourselves of them, we have no control over the automatic thoughts that pop into our heads. They are products of our negativity bias, our culture, our past (and that of our ancestors), our biology, our emotions, and the situation we're facing. Our thoughts don't make us good or bad; they are just mental events automatically pumping out of our brains in the same way that saliva is released with the smell of food. It's not personal: our thoughts don't define who or how good we are.

An essential skill in learning to work with thoughts is becoming aware of them without judging ourselves for having them, as weird and wild as they may be. One of the participants in my group started to notice that when he called his thoughts "silly" instead of "bad," he adopted a much lighter stance with them. Thoughts don't need to be taken so seriously. They're just thoughts, not the truth, and definitively not our dictator.

After we bring our thoughts into awareness, we can practice allowing them without judging ourselves for having such thoughts, because they are outside of our control. Then we can learn to see thoughts as just thoughts—as a popular bumper sticker reads, "Don't believe everything you think!"

This is where we can use a lot of our kind awareness skills, simply noticing thoughts as thoughts, as if we are standing on a mountaintop, watching different weather systems pass by. *Oh, here's a cloud of catastrophizing. Oh, and there's some jumping to conclusions to find certainty in an uncertain situation. Thanks, mind, for trying to keep me safe.* We can label our thoughts as thoughts, or even write them down to put some space and perspective between automatically believing these thoughts and seeing them simply as thoughts passing through our awareness.

Remember Russ Harris's analogy of the hotel lobby in the last chapter? Our thoughts are like customers who come into the lobby. We have no control over who arrives at our door. But we can decide who we invite upstairs—that is, which thoughts we spend time entertaining. Harris offers another analogy of thoughts being like bullies who hop on the bus as we are traveling to get somewhere. We can spend all our energy trying to boot them off the bus, or we can give them a seat away from us, even if they are unruly and speaking out of turn. The key is not to let them take over the steering and drive! We can listen to their messages to help us steer the bus—sometimes, they are providing valuable information about the obstacles on the road ahead—but we must remain in the driver's seat, evaluating their helpfulness while we keep steering the bus in line with our values and what the present environment needs.

Mindfulness teacher Joseph Goldstein describes how quickly thoughts take the wheel when we aren't aware we are having them:

> When we lose ourselves in thoughts, thoughts sweep up our
> mind and carry it away; in a very short time we can be carried
> far indeed. We hop on a train of association, not realizing that
> we have hopped on, and certainly not knowing the destination.
> Somewhere down the line, we may wake up and realize that we
> have been thinking, and that we have been taken for a ride. When
> we step down from the train, it may be in a very different state of
> mind from where we jumped aboard.

Instead, we can learn to mindfully observe our thoughts arising and passing, labeling them as just thoughts, without letting them hijack us or overstay their welcome. One helpful way of doing this is by more specifically recognizing and labeling false alarms, what cognitive therapists call *thinking traps*. These are common ways that our brains automatically jump to certainty when we are faced with uncertain situations, especially when we're activated. We can learn to notice these unhelpful habits and work backward to return to uncertainty again. As historian Daniel J. Boorstin wrote, "The greatest obstacle to discovery is not ignorance—it is the illusion of knowledge."

Here are some of the common thinking traps that we all find ourselves getting stuck in sometimes, particularly when we're activated into extreme patterns of thinking. Again, this happens automatically and completely outside our control, so we can make sure we don't start using it as another list to tell us how we're failing in life. These traps usually signal that we're activated into an emotional alarm. While we have no control over the first thought, we can decide if we want to entertain and believe it. It's simply an alarm giving us a message. Then we, as the driver of our bus, decide if it's helpful to the present situation or a false alarm based on past learning or our negativity bias.

COMMON THINKING TRAPS

ALL-OR-NOTHING THINKING *One mistake makes me/them all bad.*	**PERSONALIZATION** *If only I . . . then none of this would have happened.*
FORTUNE TELLING *It's not going to work out.*	**MIND-READING** *She looked at her phone because she's bored.*
DISQUALIFYING THE POSITIVE *You have to say that because you're my friend.*	**CATASTROPHIZING** *This symptom must mean I have cancer.*
OVERGENERALIZATION *I'm always a failure.*	**EMOTIONAL REASONING** *I feel shame, so I must be bad.*

We're not aiming for "positive" (and unrealistic) thinking; we're not changing our thoughts from *Everyone hates me* to *Everyone thinks*

I'm God's gift to the world. Instead, we're aiming for balanced thinking. We can notice, *Ah, there's all-or-nothing thinking and mind-reading
again. Thanks, mind, for trying to find certainty. I don't actually know how
others feel. Some people probably like parts of me and some people don't like
other parts of me. I can't please everyone.*

We often don't need to change our thoughts. We can change our
attitude toward our thoughts, learning to hold our thoughts gently,
seeing thoughts as just thoughts and not the truth. We realize that
thoughts are accurate signals of what emotional alarm we are in, not
what's actually happening in our environment. We learn to not believe everything we think.

Those of us with the most privilege and power question the accuracy of our own perspectives the least, often assuming dominant views
are objective or normal, rather than subjective and diverse, just like
everyone else's. As we bring our thoughts and beliefs into awareness,
we gain the ability to question these assumptions. At the same time,
we want to ensure that we're not simply replacing the false certainty
of the dominant culture with the false certainty of another narrow
version of reality on our path to creating a just and equitable collective, neglecting the complexity and numerous realities that can coexist.
Instead, we hope to move toward the humility of not knowing, with
curiosity about everyone's wide-ranging perspectives.

Staying in the gray can be uncomfortable. And yet the healthiest
way to be in the world—and the most realistic—is to acknowledge the
complexity and uncertainty of it all.

WE ALL NEED EDITORS

As a writer, I can attest that our job description is mostly editing—
reworking each sentence until it feels just right. We can give the same
attention to the sentences in our minds, too. I mentioned before how
we refer to thoughts as *the story I'm telling myself.* And as with writing,

no one expects us to produce anything close to the final product on the first go. We need multiple iterations of reflective editing. It's the same when editing our thoughts.

Cognitive therapists call this process of examining and challenging our thoughts *cognitive restructuring* and offer a huge spectrum of exercises to do so. When we wrote the curriculum for our Cognitive Behavioral Therapy Skills Group program for our Mind Space collective in BC, our workbook had pages of questions and exercises to teach participants to move from the rough drafts of automatic thoughts to more balanced and uncertain thinking. In honesty, it was an ugly mess, overwhelming participants and facilitators alike.

But then one of our facilitators stumbled upon a mnemonic that her daughter found to help teens make more skillful online comments, called THINK. We realized that all the fancy skills we were trying so unsuccessfully to summarize could be described by these few questions. We just needed to learn to talk to ourselves in the same ways we're teaching our youth to talk to each other.

The *T* stands for *true*: How true is it? In what way is our negativity bias or need for certainty influencing the accuracy of our thoughts? How can we have a more balanced, realistic—and uncertain—thought? What information are we missing? Often a missing piece of the equation is how we can cope even if the scary thing were to occur. We may be so busy trying to prevent threats from catching up to us that we don't realize how resourceful we could be if the threat were to arrive. So, rather than the first draft of *The date went horribly and she's never going to want to go out again and I will be devastated and single forever,* a truer, more balanced version could be, *There were parts of the date that didn't go well and parts that went okay. I don't know how she feels about me. If she decides not to go out again, it will hurt, and I've coped with situations like this before and been okay. Just like everyone else, I'm not for everyone.*

The *H* stands for *helpful*: How helpful is the thought? What happens if you spend time focused on this thought (giving it a room in your mind's hotel)?

The *I* is for *inspiring*: How inspiring is the thought? Would letting this thought take the steering wheel move you in the direction you want to be driving?

The *N* is for *needs*, capturing how feelings give birth to thoughts: What underlying needs is this thought signaling? Is this thought a symptom or signal that gives you valuable information about what mood or emotional state you're in? What does this information tell you about your needs right now? Maybe you need support, boundaries, self-care, or to overthrow harmful systems.

And finally, the *K* stands for *kind*, the most important question: How kind is this thought? As we know from the self-compassion research, the tone in which we relate to our inner experiences matters. How can we edit this thought with a kinder and gentler tone?

CORE BELIEFS

These kinds of exercises can be easier for more superficial automatic thoughts, like the thought you have about your partner leaving dirty dishes around. But what if we dig deeper? Cognitive therapists offer the *downward arrow* technique, where we take an automatic thought and keep asking ourselves: What does this say about me/others/the world? So, if my friend doesn't show up for our meeting, my go-to interpretation would be that she doesn't want to hang out with me. Then I ask myself again: What does that say about me? It says maybe I've hurt her or maybe she doesn't like me. And what does that say about me? That it's always my fault and I'm not worthy of belonging. I hit my core beliefs.

Core beliefs are learned patterns from our cultures, ancestors, experiences, and environment, designed to find predictability in the uncertain world we inhabit. If our automatic thoughts are playing our top ten

tracks, our core beliefs are the genre of music we always listen to. They
give the tone and tempo that influence how we interpret the world.

Yet when left in autopilot, our core beliefs keep us confined in
old stories that may no longer be true, often creating a self-fulfilling
prophecy. If our core belief is that others are uncaring, we may act in
ways that don't bring out the best in others. If our core belief is that
we aren't capable of coping, we might never put ourselves in situations
that teach us that we can cope just fine. For myself, my core belief of
not belonging led me to pretzel myself to please others so I could su-
perficially fit in, rather than show my authentic self for long enough to
feel true belonging.

While core beliefs are often more painful to hold and stubborn
to change, we can still use the same skills to cultivate more helpful
second thoughts. Remember how neuroscientists say "What fires together wires together" to explain that any thought, feeling, or action
urge that occurs over and over creates a well-trodden path in our
brains. When we notice that these automatic paths are no longer
serving us, we can start the challenging task of bushwhacking a new
one.

At the start, because our brains have never fired this way before,
it's a tough slog through thick foliage. It's hard to imagine that it will
ever be easy. But the more we keep stepping out of autopilot, bringing
awareness to our thoughts, and practicing new ways of relating to them,
the more our brains fire together in this more helpful direction, and
the smoother and easier the path in the brain becomes. With time and
practice, our autopilot can be retrained to relate more healthily to our
thoughts. Our new habits turn into the main highways of our brains.

How we relate to our thoughts can either liberate or limit us.
Sometimes, the most freeing approach is to take the power back from
our thoughts, telling them, *Thanks, mind, for trying to keep me safe with
all those scary stories. Right now, they're not very helpful, so I'm not going
to let them take the wheel.*

AN EPIDEMIC OF MISINFORMATION

A people are as healthy and confident as the stories they
tell themselves. Sick storytellers can make their nations
sick. And sick nations make for sick storytellers.

—BEN OKRI

———

A word of warning: Cognitive therapy's focus on challenging the content of our thoughts is sometimes criticized as "gaslighting therapy," because it can be misused to invalidate accurate alarms and push us away from our own inner knowing. It shares a striking resemblance to the "thought work" (*sixiang gongzue*) imposed by the Chinese state to instill ideals aligned with the political goals of the ruling party, explains cultural anthropologist Li Zhang.[7]

We're currently facing a global escalation of the use of propaganda, misinformation, and lies to gain power through brainwashing our collectives. The 2024 World Press Freedom Index reported a "worrying decline" in both media autonomy (with increased pressure from states and other political actors) and regulations to protect their integrity. "Press freedom around the world is being threatened by the very people who should be its guarantors—political authorities," they warn. "In the absence of regulation, the use of generative AI in the arsenal of disinformation for political purposes is a concern." The report adds, "Deepfakes now occupy a leading position in influencing the course of elections."

Kelly Greenhill, professor of political science at Tufts University, identifies the social conditions that breed the contagion of misinformation and lies. First, times of heightened stress, like pandemics, civic and global conflict, and polarizing politics deactivate our prefrontal cortexes, making us more susceptible to incorrect information, as we discussed already. Then, the scary lies dysregulate us even more, so we're more vulnerable to believing them. In a world that's feeling more uncertain and unsafe than ever, believing a simple conspiracy theory with conviction gives us a dopamine hit of certainty. Our thoughts don't need to be reality-based to quiet these alarms, just certain!

Then, the disruptive communication technologies of the internet are hotbeds for misinformation and lies, Greenhill explains, with the rise of new gatekeepers and presence of many actors—and well-funded bots—willing to circulate bunk. As self-interested billionaires buy up our media platforms, tinker with their algorithms and content to promote their political interests, and flood us with unregulated misinformation and lies, it's getting too easy to convince us to vote against our best interests.

We can't let the influence of the markets, politics, and nefarious actors corrupt our minds. Once we get our prefrontal cortexes back online, we can arm ourselves with the same critical thinking tools of THINK to ensure we don't let others take over the wheel of our brains. Just like we've learned to check the sources of the thoughts in our heads, we also need to assess the source of the external information we consume, including any inherent biases and conflicts of interest.

When we come across others sharing misinformation and lies, we can try nonthreatening, compassionate conversations to encourage them to keep their prefrontal cortex online, instead of defensively plunging them further into the stress response that made them so suggestible in the first place. We need to help them regulate to get their rational brains online so they can assess the accuracy for themselves. Even paying them kind attention by listening and identifying their concerns can help bring back their prefrontal cortexes.

Debunking should avoid repeating the misinformation, which can unintentionally further cement it because of the *illusory truth effect* that makes us believe false information just from repeated exposure to it. Instead, we need to repeat the true information from a variety of sources that people trust. We can help each other explore how these beliefs developed, what sources were explored, and what potential interests may be fueling these sources. The research of Cornell University's behavior scientist Gordon Pennycook and others shows that getting participants to just think about how accurate a news piece is improves their discrimination of what content they later share. Similarly, asking probing questions to make people reflect on a news article—and thus slowing them down—improves resistance to misinformation.

James Baldwin said, "If I love you, I have to make you conscious of the things you don't see." Sometimes, that's a very uncomfortable task. But it's even more distressing when members of our collective willingly harm ourselves and each other. Love is continuing to care for each other even when we're wrong.

That sweet girl from my son's preschool will eventually learn that an invitation to a nature walk with new friends will likely be less awkward if she doesn't show up naked. While she might be distressed when she learns that she misunderstood, this new information will make her life easier in the long run.

"It's painful to learn the truth," said Gabor Maté of his journey to overcome past conditioning from living under different political regimes. "But I'd rather be disillusioned than illusioned."

INCHING TOWARD REVOLUTION

Historian and activist Rebecca Solnit says revolutions are not fast, linear, spontaneous leaps forward. Instead, they are like a mushroom sprouting out of the ground after a rain—as if from nowhere, but originating from the foundation of a vast, organized underground network. Changes in our thinking seem insignificant, she says, until very different outcomes emerge from transformed assumptions about who and what matters.

Yet holding hope for a better future is not only about how we think. "Hope is not like a lottery ticket you can sit on the sofa and clutch, feeling lucky," says Solnit in *Hope in the Dark*.[8] "Hope is an axe you break down doors with in an emergency. Hope just means another world might be possible, not promised, not guaranteed. Hope calls for action."

NINE

TAKING BACK THE REINS

Action is the antidote to despair.

—Joan Baez

———

AFTER YEARS OF STUDYING THE DEPTHS OF PSYCHOLOGY, I STUMBLED ACROSS A STUDY that surprised me. It showed that simply scheduling a coffee date or a walk outside, even when you don't feel like it, is just as effective as our sophisticated psychotherapies for improving symptoms of depression.[1] I searched the literature, desperately trying to disprove it. But other studies supported its conclusions.[2] We really can change how we feel by changing how we act.

Yet it's hard to change our behaviors. The biggest challenge isn't in knowing what's healthiest for both ourselves and our collective; it's implementing it. How many times have we made resolutions to adopt healthier habits or vowed to never engage in unhelpful ones ever again, only to chastise ourselves for failing? Then the waves of distress arising from not meeting these expectations lead us to engage even more in the unhealthy behavior in attempts to soothe the awful feeling (what's known as the *abstinence violation effect*).

While changing behaviors can offer fast results, we still must compassionately understand all the obstacles that drive our behavior—our feelings, thoughts, past and present relationships, and environments— which we discussed in previous chapters. There's never a quick fix to complex challenges.

One stumbling block with behavior change is that we usually don't feel like doing it, especially when our emotional alarms give us unhelpful messages that are more about our negativity bias or needs of the past than the current situation in front of us. We can also struggle with acting in unhelpful ways when we've been conditioned to switch our primary emotions into more comfortable secondary ones, like anger or shame, so the emotion is no longer pushing us to act in ways that match the needs of the situation. And sometimes, we're simply too activated or shut down to act skillfully at all.

Adding to the challenge, our emotions are designed to address the short-term threats and rewards in front of us, not the nuances of each action's long-term consequences within complex systems, which require the slower path of consulting our prefrontal cortex. For this reason, we need to ask ourselves, *Is this emotion's action urge helpful in the long run?*

We can start by exploring what action urges accompany each emotion. Here's a chart of some common action urges. We've all been conditioned by different cultures and histories, and we are neurodiverse in our biology, so this may look different for you.

We can then add in each emotion's action urge to our emotion charts, just like we did with thoughts and body sensations.

EMOTIONS PUSH FOR ACTION

EMOTION	POTENTIAL MESSAGES IT'S SIGNALING	POSSIBLE ACTIONS IT'S MOTIVATING
JOY/LUST/ LOVE	Reward Present	Approach Savor Share Cherish Repeat
ANGER	Boundary violation Reward blocked Injustice	Assert Confront Protect
FEAR	Threat Uncertainty	Avoid Prepare
SADNESS	Loss of something important Not enough rewards present	Mourn Seek support Replace what's lost Hibernate until rewards return Try a more rewarding approach or environment
GUILT	Actions caused harm	Show accountability Repair or make amends
SHAME	People are rejecting a part of you	Find and build safer spaces/communities Hide parts of self from unsafe people who can't be trusted with them
ENVY	Someone else has rewards you want	Find similar reward for yourself
JEALOUSY	Threat of reward being taken by someone else	Cherish, express gratitude, and protect the relationship/rewards you already have
DISGUST	Observing something you perceive as toxic, immoral, or unwanted	Avoid Expunge

FOR EACH EMOTION LISTED BELOW, ANSWER THE FOLLOWING QUESTIONS:

- What types of situations typically induce this signal?
- Body Sensations: What do you feel in your body as you scan the different parts?
    - What's the temperature of different areas?
    - What areas feel more tight or more loose?
    - What areas feel more heavy or more light?
    - Is there any movement in any areas (such as shaking, pulsing, tingling)?
- Automatic Thoughts: What do you believe about yourself (such as your worth or ability to cope), others, the world?
- What is the potential message of the emotion?
- Action Urges:
    - Does it feel like your body is being pushed to act in any certain way?
    - Does it feel like your body is being pushed to adopt a certain posture, tone of voice, or facial expression?

Joy

_____

Anger

_____

Fear

_____

Sadness

_____

Guilt

_____

Shame

_____

There are many other emotions you can explore in the same way. You can try observing your signatures for the other emotional signals you typically encounter, such as jealousy, envy, love, or disgust.

RESPONDING WITH SKILLFUL ACTIONS

When we notice an emotional alarm arise within us, we can put together all the skills we've been learning in the other chapters to help us respond with the most helpful action. This exercise is adapted from dialectical behavioral therapy, such as Marsha Linehan's *DBT Skills Training Manual* and Christine Dunkley's *Regulating Emotion the DBT Way*.

I. STEP OUT OF AUTOPILOT and pay attention to what's happening in this moment:
   A. What state of activation are you in?
      1. Do you need time to help bring your system back into balance so you can respond most skillfully?
      2. As needed, seek safety and try practicing kind attention, grounding, regulation skills, validation, and co-regulation.
   B. What emotion is present?
      1. What message is it telling you?
         a. Is this an accurate assessment of the current situation or a false alarm responding to your negativity bias or past/historical threats?
         b. How does it show up in your body? Can you practice acceptance and allowing skills with these body sensations rather than pushing them away or thinking about the emotion?
      2. What action urge is connected to this emotion (i.e., how is it pushing you to act)?
         a. Is this the primary emotion's action urge (that matches the present situation), or are you in a secondary emotion (that is leading you astray)?

3. Will acting on this emotion's action urge at the current intensity and time be helpful in the long run?

a. If the emotion's action urge intensity matches the needs of the situation, embody it and act on the urge.

b. If a more intense emotional reaction would be more skillful (for example, you've harmed someone and it would be helpful to express more guilt—instead of indifference—to push you to be accountable and repair appropriately; or you've suppressed your anger, so you need to express more of its action urge to protect yourself from violation or injustice):

(1) Practice embodying the primary emotion's features by changing your posture to mimic that of the helpful emotion. (for example, cower down for guilt, or puff up for anger).

(2) Act in line with the action urge of the helpful emotion (for example, apologize for guilt, or assert healthy boundaries for resentment).

c. If a less intense or delayed emotional reaction would be more skillful (for example, it's more helpful to wait until a better time, place, or person to express the emotion's action urge, or to decrease the intensity of the emotion's action urge to better match the needs of the situation):

(1) Practice embodying the opposite of the unhelpful emotion urge's features (or that of a different, more helpful emotion, such as the primary emotion if you're stuck in a secondary emotion) by changing your posture to mimic the opposite of the unhelpful emotion urge (for example, cower down in unhelpful anger urge, or stand tall in unhelpful shame or guilt urge).

(2) Choose alternative actions that oppose the unhelpful action urge (for example, if anger urge to fight is unhelpful in a situation, move away instead; if shame urge to hide is unhelpful in a situation, practice sharing this part of yourself with someone who is safe to hold it).

STEP 1
Temperature Check: Where are you on the emotional dial?

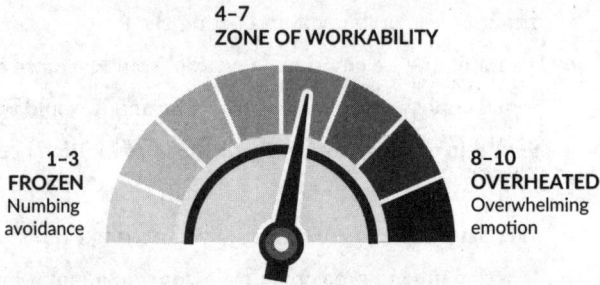

4–7
ZONE OF WORKABILITY

1–3
FROZEN
Numbing
avoidance

8–10
OVERHEATED
Overwhelming
emotion

STEP 2
Practice skills to regulate if needed
(e.g., ABC's, DIAL, Grounding)

STEP 3
Investigate emotion's message and urge

STEP 4
Assess how much of emotion's expression is helpful in this situation

STEP 5
Respond skillfully

<< NEED MORE	JUST RIGHT	NEED LESS >>
If **MORE** emotional activation or urge would be helpful	Be mindful of emotion	If **LESS** urge would be helpful
Embody emotion's features	Express emotion as is helpful	Change bodily expression
Act in line with helpful urges	Act in line with helpful urges	Act opposite or choose an alternative action

Adapted from Christine Dunkley's *Regulating Emotion the DBT Way*.

EMOTION	POTENTIAL INSTINCTIVE POSTURE	POTENTIAL ACTION URGE		POTENTIAL ALTERNATIVE POSTURE	POTENTIAL ACTION URGE
Anger	Tense muscles Clenched fists & jaw	Approach Conform Fight	If the action urge is not helpful right now (or too much), try an alternative	Loosen muscles Relax face & smile slightly Relax hands	Gently avoid what is angering you Practice empathy Be kind (even a little, to anyone)
Fear	Closed posture Tense muscles Eyes, chin, shoulders down	Avoid Flee Freeze		Relax muscles consciously Eyes & ears open Confident posture	Approach what causes fear Baby steps, support
Sadness	Downcast reserved posture	Withdraw Decrease activity		Upbeat posture Relaxed face, gentle smile	Become active Baby steps Connect with others
Guilt	Closed posture Quiet, gentle, speech Soft gaze	Apologize Make amends		Eye contact Proud posture	Be assertive Empathize but don't apologize
Shame	Downcast gaze Small, closed posture	Hide		Eye contact Proud posture	Self-compassion Tell the shameful thing to people who will accept you

Adapted from Marsha Linehan's *DBT Skills Training Manual.*

For example, we may notice a surge of anger arising during a meeting. We can first assess where we are on the emotional dial to see if we need to practice any skills to help us get our prefrontal cortex online so we have the capacity to reflect on the experience. Then, we can identify that anger is here and get curious as to what it's trying to signal to us. We might notice that it's telling us that there's an injustice happening right now in the meeting. Or we might notice that the emotion is secondary, so we can get curious as to what the primary one is. Perhaps we were just told that our actions caused harm, and we realize that we switched the uncomfortable experience of guilt into the more tolerable secondary emotion of anger. Or we might notice that our anger alarm is ringing because something in the meeting—perhaps a mannerism or the tone of voice of the speaker—reminds us of someone who harmed us in the past, so this current emotional alarm is signaling a historical threat rather than a present one. Regardless of the meaning of the signal, we can practice our skills of surfing the wave of anger by noticing and allowing all the sensations of anger in our bodies with compassion.

We can then reflect on whether this emotion's action urge is helpful right now in the meeting. If it's signaling a present injustice, we may decide that it's most skillful to speak up to protect others or fix the problem. We might decide to embody the anger's signature, such as sitting up tall, speaking firmly, and taking up space in the meeting to ensure that this issue is addressed. Or if we notice that the anger is secondary to our primary emotion of guilt, we may decide that the most helpful response is to embody the guilt's signature, by speaking softer, releasing our tense muscles, taking accountability for the harm we've caused, and making efforts to repair and learn from it. In the situation where the anger links to a historical alarm, we may engage in the opposite actions of anger to help calm the signal, such as adopting a softer, gentle posture, moving our attention away from the person who's activating us, and practicing empathy and acts of kindness toward those in the meeting.

Similarly, if we notice sadness and low mood, we can first check where we are on the dial of activation and practice skills to get our prefrontal cortex back online if needed. We can feel all the sensations in the body to help us allow and be with the uncomfortable emotion with compassion, without making it worse with attempts to push it away or ruminate about it. Then we can ask ourselves what this emotional alarm is trying to communicate to us. We may notice that it's signaling that we've experienced a loss that requires tenderness. Or we may notice that it's signaling low rewards, because we've been stuck in a cycle of isolating and inactivity for too long.

Then we can ask ourselves what would be the most helpful response in the long run. In the situation where we are grieving a loss, we may decide that it's most helpful to give ourselves space to feel and process the loss by stepping away from our responsibilities so we can rest, nurture ourselves, and seek support, recovering our resources to eventually find and rebuild what we've lost. If we're noticing we've withdrawn at home for too long, and it's no longer serving us, we can work to engage in the opposite of the low mood's action urge, by activating with increased activity and social connection. We can start by changing our posture to the opposite of the low mood and sadness. Instead of looking down and making ourselves small, we can stand tall, with our shoulders back, and look up or forward. We can see if practicing a relaxed half-smile helps to enliven us.

Behavioral activation for depression includes scheduling activities that achieve a sense of agency, connection, and structure or engage our seeking, care, lust, and play systems. Even though we don't feel like it, we might start with small, manageable steps to socialize, by scheduling a short walk or phone call with a friend. We can watch a comedy, dance, or play a game or sport to induce pleasure. Or we may clean a few dishes or help someone with a task to restore our sense of agency. We can especially try to seek out activities that matter to us, reconnecting us with our purpose.

I must emphasize that I'm not teaching us to stop feeling by offering these techniques. Most of us need to feel *more*. But by learning to be more in control of our emotion-fueled actions, we can build confidence in holding and expressing emotions skillfully, instead of getting hijacked by them. Then we can use their fire to address the problems we face.

USING THE COMPASS OF OUR VALUES

I am publishing this book into a world where many people and groups will likely reject me. I'm not for everyone, nor could I ever be. My shame alarm is blaring, ramped up by the historical alarms of my past conditioning. Shame tells me to hide the parts of myself that could be rejected, or to only share them with the people that I know are safe enough to hold them. And I'm overriding its warning.

I anticipate that shame will be a recurrent visitor as this book comes out. And it will be distressing. But these evolutionary alarms can't see the bigger picture of the purpose we choose for ourselves. My core values are connection, contribution, and compassion, so if this book has any potential to bring more unity and kindness into the world, even if just to a few people, it's worth the pain of all the shame that might come along with living a life that matters to me.

When we feel the storms of emotional alarms, whether they're alerting us to past or present threats and rewards, we need a compass to keep us moving in our chosen direction. When researchers studied the people of Okinawa, Japan, whose women lived longer than any others around the world, they identified the community's philosophy of *ikigai*—finding one's purpose—as a secret to their longevity. Japanese psychotherapist and Zen Buddhist Shoma Morita created the value-oriented therapy centered in *ikigai*, Morita therapy, which teaches us to mindfully accept our feelings while working to change our actions to align with our purpose.[3] Morita taught that everyone has a purpose, although sometimes it takes patience to find it.

When our environments or actions don't align with our values and purpose, we suffer. For example, in her memoir *Crying in the Bathroom*, Erika L. Sánchez explains how sick she became when working for a PR firm, despite its rewarding salary. She stopped sleeping, lost weight, withdrew from loved ones, struggled to function, and thought of suicide. As the policies and practices of the job were demeaning and controlling, Sánchez's blaring threat alarms signaled an important message: this environment was both unsafe and unrewarding.

"I was afraid to tell my mom I had quit the highest-paying job I'd ever had, but once I did, she was relieved rather than disappointed," Sánchez wrote. Despite the job paying far beyond the factory wages of her parents who'd immigrated from Mexico, her mom responded, "Tú, si eres chingona" ("You're a badass bitch"). A couple of weeks later, Sánchez took a new job consulting for a project in Trinidad, interviewing low-income women to report on the life-saving procedures of cervical cancer screening. "As I stood in the passport line waiting to enter the country, I remembered that only a few weeks before, I was sobbing on my couch, wanting to die," Sánchez wrote. "And now here I was in a foreign land, not only functioning but exhilarated by my circumstances." The compass of following her purpose brought wellness to Sánchez in a way that financial success couldn't.

Living by your values may seem like a privilege that only a lucky few get to practice. We may feel that we must adopt the values of others to survive or fit in, without questioning if they serve us well. And too often, we're jumping from fire to fire without much time to notice what direction we're heading in. When we're simply trying to make rent or keep our family safe, it may feel frivolous to consider our values. Yet in *Man's Search for Meaning*, physician Viktor Frankl documented how his focus on purpose provided the compass he needed to survive the torturous conditions as a prisoner of the concentration camps that killed his wife, brother, father, and mother. "Those who have a 'why' to live for, can bear with almost any 'how,'" he wrote, referencing Nietzsche. Even when the world around us steals our freedom in a myriad of ways, we can empower ourselves from within by living by our chosen values.

FINDING WHAT MATTERS TO YOU

We all hold unique values that describe how we want to relate to the world, other people, and ourselves. And that's wonderful. Remember, the healthiest systems depend on having many diverse parts that function differently yet together.

The list of potential values is long, including many we've never even considered. Here's a short sampling, but you can explore ones that fit best with what matters most to you:

Acceptance	Freedom
Accountability	Generosity
Adaptability	Gratitude
Adventure	Honesty
Ambition	Humility
Authenticity	Inclusion
Balance	Industry
Beauty	Integrity
Belonging	Intimacy
Caring	Justice
Compassion	Kindness
Connection	Leadership
Contribution/Legacy	Learning/Growth
Community	Love
Courage	Loyalty
Creativity	Mindfulness
Curiosity	Obedience
Dependability	Open-mindedness
Dignity	Order
Discipline	Patience
Duty	Peacefulness
Empowerment	Persistence
Equality	Reciprocity
Fairness	Respect
Faith	Responsibility
Flexibility	Security/Protection

Self-awareness	Supportiveness
Sensuality	Sustainability
Spirituality	Tradition
Stability	Wisdom

Values differ from goals in that values describe *how* we globally act and relate to the world, not *what* we are specifically achieving in discrete contexts. Goals can be completed and checked off, while values are always available to us as our compass to direct ongoing actions. If you value compassion and retire from your helping profession, you can approach your other relationships and community with the same care. Or if you no longer have time to express creativity in the formal pursuits you did before having children, you can use this value to guide how you work or parent.

Many forms of therapy offer practices to help us discover or clarify our values. This exercise is an adaptation of acceptance and commitment therapy's (ACT) *magic wand* exercise:[4]

Imagine you have a magic wand that removes all the obstacles and difficulties in your life so that you no longer have to consider any of these challenges:

1. HOW do you want to live your life?

2. WHAT does a full and meaningful life look like to you?

3. WHAT is most important to you?

4. WHAT qualities do you want to cultivate?

5. HOW would you want to show up and behave?

6. HOW do you want to be in your relationships with others?

Now imagine it's your ideal ninetieth birthday party. Two or three people whom you really care about make speeches about what you stand for, how you have contributed, what you mean to them, and the role you play in the world.

7. IN your ideal life, where you have acted in alignment with the values you wish to practice, what would you hear them saying?

We may notice grief arising with this exercise as we notice the gap between how we're currently living and what we value. We can gently hold the discomfort by offering ourselves compassion, surfing the sensations in the body, and then listening to their message. Remember how grief is a helpful signal that tells us what truly matters to us. Because there are so many qualities on the list of values that may sound important in our heads, the powerful emotion of grief helps us identify what we value most in our hearts. In the same way, we may notice the emotional signal of gratitude arise when we've landed on important values that we're already living by.

We often add second arrows of criticizing ourselves whenever we aren't able to practice all our chosen values all the time. Instead, we can hold our values lightly, because we may need to prioritize different values in different seasons of life. But they're always there as a compass when we need them. While I hold creativity and adventure as values, when I'm overstretched in high-stress periods, I lean more on my core values of compassion and connection, knowing that the other values will always be there waiting for me when I have more capacity to practice them.

Values also differ from emotional states, like happiness. "Happiness cannot be pursued. It must ensue," Viktor Frankl explained. "One must have a reason to 'be happy.'" If we act in ways that embody our values, we will experience more pleasant emotions, even when we're experiencing adversity. When we mistake happiness as a value, we can instead identify our underlying values by asking: How would I be

showing up if I were happy? What would matter to me? How would
I be living?

FROM OUR VALUES EXPLORATION with the magic wand, we can list three
values that matter most:

_____

_____

_____

WE ALSO CAN CONSIDER core areas of life that are important to us (such
as relationships, school, work, volunteering/service, community,
spirituality/religion, leisure, health, or any other areas that feel
important):

_____

_____

_____

THEN WE CAN CONSIDER which area of our life is the highest priority
right now and what values from our list may best act as our
compass to help us move in the direction that matters most in
this area.

_____

_____

_____

From this exercise, we can identify specific areas that we might want to prioritize for improvement. For example, if I notice that I've been showing less compassion toward myself and others at work—perhaps I'm burned out and operating on autopilot—I may choose to prioritize compassion practices during my work hours.

Once we've found an area to work on that matters to us, we can then practice goal setting. Here's a value-oriented version of SMART goals adapted by Russ Harris in *ACT Made Simple*:[5]

SMART GOALS

Specific: What exact actions will you take? When, where, and possibly with whom will you take them?

Measurable: Ensure your goal is measurable (e.g., *Practice self-compassion break twice a day during work*) instead of a vague concept (e.g., *Be more compassionate at work*).

Attainable: Rate how confident you are on a scale of zero to ten. If your confidence is less than eight on the scale, break the goal into several smaller, more realistic goals.

Relevant: Ensure your goal is guided by your values and the domain of life that's important to you.

Time-bound: Set a realistic date and time for completing the goal. If we say we're going to do it for all of eternity, we can feel overwhelmed and lose motivation. Starting with short time periods allows us to feel a sense of mastery when we achieve our goal. (I often like to start with the smallest goal I can attain in the shortest amount of time, to build my confidence.)

Sometimes, we set goals or hope to develop new behaviors, only to find that no matter how hard we try, we can't achieve them. While we often blame or shame ourselves and others when we can't stick to the ideal behaviors we hope for, we aren't bad or lazy. We're often suffering from the simple math of the rewards not outweighing the costs. So much of the time, our behaviors are reinforced by things we aren't even aware of, because we're all entangled in complex systems where our individual behaviors create cascades in multiple relationships and feedback loops. For example, when we try to assert boundaries, prioritize balance, or advocate for justice and equity, these changes may affect other people in our system who may try to push us back to the status quo. Or when we choose healthier behaviors, our partners or families may feel envy, jealousy, or guilt because they haven't changed their behaviors in the same way or don't like that we're spending more time away from them. We might not consciously link this new tension in our relationships to our new behaviors, but we're still implicitly registering them as costs of behavior change.

Our behaviors can be reinforced or weakened by applying reinforcement or punishment, whether we're aware of it or not. Behaviors may be positively reinforced by rewarding us with more positive things (such as receiving praise or improving the sense of connection in our relationships or communities). Or they can be negatively reinforced by removing negative things (such as feeling less anxiety or having less tension in a relationship). Behaviors can also be punished by taking away rewards (such as stopping contact with someone) or adding costs (such as criticizing them).

Psychology research shows that reinforcement is exceedingly more effective, fast, and enduring than punishment, because it's more motivating and keeps us regulated and out of the shame, blame, resentment, and revenge that punishment often induces.[6] Intermittent rewards—such as with gambling—are the most reinforcing. So, if you can't figure out why you keep going back to that slot machine of an avoidant ex who only shows you love once in a while, the power of intermittent reinforcement may be to blame.

We can also extinguish a behavior when a response is no longer reinforced (for example, if we don't react to someone's acts of affection or antagonism, we no longer reinforce these behaviors, and they will typically cease). Of note, when we try to extinguish a behavior, we usually first notice an *extinction burst*, where the behavior actually gets bigger in attempts to achieve the previously reinforced reaction. For example, when my children react to each other's taunting, they reinforce the behavior, so they're more likely to repeat it. However, if one ignores the other's taunts, the other may first taunt louder (the *extinction burst*) to try to get the old reaction. But if he continues to ignore (and thus not reinforce) the taunting, the other will usually stop the unhelpful behavior because there's no longer a reward for doing it.

This strategy only works when there isn't egregious harm that needs to be immediately prevented with firmer actions. We can choose for ourselves whether a situation requires us to expend the energy to fight for hard boundaries on what behavior's not okay or whether we can more passively extinguish it.

When we're struggling to follow through with our goals, we can consider all the costs and benefits influencing what behaviors we adopt, an exercise used in *Motivational Interviewing*, developed by William R. Miller and Stephen Rollnick. As we fill out this table, we can pay particular attention to the subtle reinforcement or punishment patterns, with both short-term and long-term impacts.

	BENEFITS	COSTS
STAYING THE SAME		
CHANGING BEHAVIOR		

If you've filled out all the boxes and feel overwhelmed by all the information, you can circle around three of the points from any box that most align with your values. Then you can use this information to help you decide whether the benefits of changing this behavior outweigh the costs. A lot of the time, this exercise validates that there are a lot of costs to behavior change, so we don't have to blame and shame ourselves for struggling to follow through. Perhaps it's not the right time and place, or perhaps it's not in alignment with our own values. This exercise isn't about convincing yourself to change. It's about accepting reality and truly assessing what behaviors are helpful for you to choose right now.

If we do want to change the behavior to align with our chosen direction, we can look at changing our reinforcement patterns so there are more benefits and fewer costs. Until that balance is in the behavior's favor, it will be unsustainable to continue. For example, you may want to increase your physical activity because health is a value to you. But if starting an exercise routine is making you more isolated and removed from your loved ones, and connection is your core value, is there a way to adapt how you exercise to make it an activity done with those you love? Or if you're trying to commit more time to a community movement, but your partner is complaining that you're not at home enough anymore, can you explore options together of having them join in, or offer higher quality time when you are together?

A TRIAL-AND-ERROR LIFE

Fall seven times, stand up eight.

—Japanese Proverb

We can't heal by only feeling better in a sick world. We need to make a better world through actions that fix its problems. As we spin around in the storm of all the world's moving parts, we can use the compass of our values to take small steps toward our purpose.

But change is hard, messy, slow, and fickle. We try, mess up, repair, and try again. We push too hard, burn out, rest up, and try again. We focus too much on others, retreat, find balance, then try again.

Life is a constant practice of trial and error. Sometimes, our best efforts at progress backfire, because they have unintended consequences on the larger systems we inhabit. What worked yesterday may no longer work for the new world we've arrived in today. As every part of our system keeps changing, and each change impacts every other part of the system, nobody has it all figured out. Because tomorrow will offer a completely new world to adapt to once again.

If you haven't yet cemented perfect habits despite trying desperately for decades, then maybe you're healthier than you think. We're functioning best when we have flexible responses to meet each new situation, not fixed and narrow habits that solved the challenges of yesterday—or 1984. Yes, consistency is helpful by offering a taste of certainty in our constantly shifting world. And also, we can learn to step out of autopilot and master the process of paying kind attention to our current experiences. Then we can dial up or down our emotions' urges to meet each new situation with the unique actions they require.

Luckily, we're well-equipped to navigate this landscape. With our GPS of emotional alarms to locate the threats and rewards, our prefrontal cortex to interpret what's helpful in the long run, and our compass of values to show us the way, we can stay fast on our feet to solve the problems we face, one small step at a time. Especially when we do so together.

TEN

STAYING IN CONNECTION

The strongest among us are those who can reach for others.

—SUE JOHNSON

———————

I WORKED AS A LIFEGUARD IN MY TEENS AND TWENTIES AT THE UNIVERSITY POOL. MANY of the shifts were coupled with aquacise classes, and I needed work, so I played the extroverted aerobics instructor who danced around the busy pool deck to pay the bills.

When I was promoted to supervisor, I received my very own golden keys to the facility, which granted me permission to swim alone in the massive, Olympic-sized pools after hours, where I was spoiled by the space and freedom of the wide-open lanes. When my best friend joined me, we finished our midnight swims by blasting the music to overpower the beats coming from the crammed nightclub next door. Surrounded by the solitude of the empty facility, we danced and laughed and sang while balancing precariously on our floating pool mats, savoring these precious moments of separation from the crowds and chaos of the world.

Fast-forward twenty years, and I found myself in the exact same position, this time with my family, in a completely empty facility. But it felt entirely different. A huge wave of grief and panic overtook my body as I grasped my kickboard, floating in the stillness of isolation once again.

It was 2020. We'd waited many weeks to get this one turn at our community center's pool, because we were only permitted to swim with our household's small bubble. Primed by months of social distancing and Covid restrictions, my sensitized separation alarm wouldn't settle down. As I scanned the empty pool, I couldn't stop comparing the experience to the past decade of swimming there as smiling children and chatting seniors crowded the space. While I'd hoped that returning to the pool would bring back a sense of normalcy, it only reminded me further of what we had lost: our connection to each other. Despite previously identifying as an introvert, the pandemic created a social hunger I'd never experienced before. I became obsessed with seeking connection to soothe me, with my separation alarm in overdrive whenever I spent time alone.

Remember, we have three subcortical alarm systems that keep us safe: fear to alert us to threats to our safety and certainty, anger to alert us to threats to our agency and justice, and separation distress to alert us to threats to bonding and belonging. When people come in to see me with surface symptoms of anxiety, panic, self-harm, depression, addictions, or suicidality, as we explore what specific alarms are sounding and why, it's often the separation alarm that's underlying their intolerable distress.

We already explored how we've evolved to fear abandonment and rejection as a survival advantage. "Togetherness is the most defining feature of human beings," genomics researcher Steve Cole told me as I grappled with my own separation distress during the pandemic. "This is the reason we don't get eaten by all kinds of things bigger, better, and stronger than us. The flip side is that if you are fundamentally a togetherness-based organism and you suddenly lack togetherness, you're about as naked and dead as possible. You're going to get eaten," he explained. "The thing to know about loneliness is it's a surprisingly strong danger signal for the human brain."

Solitude can nourish us for brief periods of time when we're securely attached to others with regular contact or reminders of our belonging, as it did in the empty pool prior to the pandemic. When we've had enough experiences of co-regulation with others, especially in early life, we can learn to self-soothe in their absence and enjoy these moments to ourselves. But without this co-regulating care in either our present or early life environments, periods of solitude can induce a frantic panic to reestablish connection, or a crash into despair when we can't find it. Our evolutionary alarm screams, *Danger: You've strayed too far. Go back and find the safety of your group!*

I grew up in Vancouver, a city known for its opioid crisis. In medical school, I volunteered on weekends at a health clinic in the Downtown Eastside, a neighborhood with the highest rates of the intersecting social problems of addictions, poverty, homelessness, and mental health conditions in the city. It also has more people living alone and disconnected from society than any other part of town.[1]

One of Vancouver's researchers, Bruce Alexander, a psychologist and professor emeritus at Simon Fraser University, conducted the famous "Rat Park" experiments in the 1970s and '80s to study the psychology of addictions.[2] When he separated rats to live alone and offered them both water and cocaine, the rats compulsively chose the drug until they overdosed and died. But when he housed rats together in a "rat park," free to play, socialize, and mate with one another, they chose to drink water over cocaine. When they did take a sip of the cocaine-laced liquid, they did so in moderation and never overdosed. They only struggled with the dangerous consumption of drugs when disconnected from others.

During my psychiatry training, I spent five years on an isolating infertility journey before I was lucky enough to start my own family. During that time of surgeries and interventions, I required admission to the hospital for a complication. As I lay in my sterile bed the first night in the emergency room, alone and scared, the nurse gave me an IV opioid for the pain. In that moment, I understood addictions in a way my years of schooling could never teach me. A blanket of warmth overtook me, as if a roomful of loved ones were hugging me and holding my hand. Within seconds, I no longer felt my separation alarm sounding. It's no surprise we saw opioid overdoses rise by

60 percent and substance use by 25 percent during the isolation of the pandemic.[3]

Chronic separation from others—whether its alarms are felt in frustration, panic, grief, shame, or loneliness—is not just uncomfortable, it's a leading risk factor for death. It exceeds the health risks associated with obesity, inactivity, excessive drinking, air pollution, and smoking over fifteen cigarettes a day, according to a 2010 review of 148 studies led by researchers Julianne Holt-Lunstad and Timothy Smith from Brigham Young University.[4] Their study found a 50 percent increased likelihood for all-around survival for people with stronger social ties.

"It was this study that really opened our eyes to how very real a problem this is," Smith told me as we discussed his study. "This is way more important than anything we possibly imagined. And it's been so neglected over the years," he said. Smith's research showed that it's not only the feelings of separation distress that hurt our health. It's the actual size and quality of our social network that determines our risk of future illness and premature death, even if we're not distressed about it. "We can't just alter loneliness; we need to also change our social networks," he told me. So, even if you're quite content with going it alone, or you've numbed the alarm so you no longer feel it, your body is impacted just the same by the harms of social isolation.

We've already explored how our body's alarm systems aren't that specific. Nor are they adapted to modern society. No matter which subcortical alarm system is activated—whether fear, anger, or separation distress—the signals push our bodies to get ready for an attack from a predator's wounding injury, ramping up inflammation while sacrificing immune function. As our alarms monitor our environment for threats, they sound when they sense that we've been separated for too long, sending our cells into this stress response, whether we're listening to the alarms or not.

These alarm systems are meant to be short-term solutions, with our body returning to its natural balance once we've overcome the disruption. But when the problem of isolation is ongoing, this constant activation of our stress signaling not only makes us feel bad, but it dysregulates our immune systems in ways that make us vulnerable to inflammatory-mediated conditions such as heart disease, Alzheimer's, cancer, depression, and many others, as we discussed in Chapter Three.

Luckily, we all have the capacity to reestablish our belonging to our collective, even when we're not born or married into connection.

A SOCIAL FIX

The summer I separated from my co-parent, I picked up Mia Birdsong's book, *How We Show Up*, to help us navigate the tough transition. As the founding executive director of Next River, a culture change lab for interconnected freedom, Birdsong describes herself as a family activist and futurist who has spent decades proposing new visions of who and how we can be with each other.

Birdsong explains that the American Dream of individuality, with its narrow focus on an insular nuclear family to meet all our needs, has left us lonely, disconnected, and miserable. "In response to the fear and discomfort we feel, we've built walls, and instead of leaning on one another, we find ourselves leaning on concrete," she writes. "We've forgotten the key element that helped us make progress in the first place: community."

Birdsong encourages us to expand our concept of family to include more love, inclusion, and mutual support, envisioning a sense of interconnectedness that includes the much wider network of community around us. "Our work is to become more aware of what's already there and peel back the delusion of separateness," Birdsong teaches. "We can attune ourselves to opportunities to come closer instead of stay isolated, to reach out instead of do nothing, to say, 'I'm here! Come play with me, come know me, come let me see you.'"

Many researchers confirm that these more expansive ways of creating social connection can halt the dangerous inflammatory cascade of isolation in our bodies. Smith and Holt-Lunstad's team followed up their 2010 study with another review of 106 high-quality studies in

2021. They found that even brief social interventions can prolong life when we're sick, to the same extent as cardiac rehab, diet, and exercise.[5]

It's not just immune function and inflammation that shift with social contact. The hormone oxytocin is released when mothers breastfeed and care for their babies to promote attachment and confidence. It's also released with all kinds of social bonding, especially those that involve touch, support, compassion, or care. Many studies show that oxytocin helps regulate stress (reducing blood pressure and cortisol levels), reduce anxiety, increase pain thresholds, and promote healing.[6]

We don't need a soul mate, household of best friends, or tight-knit family to gain the benefits of a social cure. Even informal, casual interactions with acquaintances and strangers—called *weak ties*—can be just as effective in restoring our sense of well-being and belonging as intimate connections with loved ones. Gillian Sandstrom, a researcher at the University of Essex, found that while the number of interactions with *strong ties* (such as family and close friends) improved people's sense of well-being and belonging, "the same was true of the weak tie interactions"—relationships involving less-frequent contact, low emotional intensity, and limited intimacy (such as greeting a stranger on the street).[7] Sandstrom had participants count their number of interactions as they went through their days. They reported greater subjective well-being and sense of belonging on days when they had more weak tie interactions.

In another part of her study, she measured how many interactions students had with classmates. Those who had the most interactions, regardless of whether they had any friends in the class, reported greater subjective feelings of happiness and belonging. In another of Sandstrom's studies, people even reported that chatting with the barista at a coffee shop led to a greater sense of belonging and happiness.[8] In a different large study, Sandstrom's team found that people perceive a quick smile, greeting, or chat as an act of kindness toward them, with both parties reporting greater life satisfaction with even these tiny moments of connection.[9] This echoes the work of Sandstrom's collaborator Elizabeth Dunn, a psychology professor at the University of British Columbia, whose study showed that participants reported feeling greater well-being than expected when interacting with a stranger, equivalent to the mood boost they experienced when interacting with their romantic partner.[10]

"Weak ties are so important, and yet, it feels like we underestimate them," Sandstrom told me. "We have so many more of them than we have strong ties, and they're so much easier to build. And they can do a good job in filling in gaps."

We often don't take advantage of these potential health boosters when we cross paths with each other. "I think people are so focused on efficiency that they're losing out on these moments of connection and maybe not even realizing they are doing it," Sandstrom said. "Each individual conversation with a stranger or weak tie isn't necessarily anything special, but they add up to something which is even more important: a sense of trust and community."

Yet chatting up a stranger can feel scary. Sandstrom's research found that most people's hesitancy relates to their worries about their own conversational enjoyment and ability, how likable they are, and how enjoyable the other person will find the experience.[11] However, she found that these fears were "massively inaccurate" and "vastly overblown," as people's conversational enjoyment, abilities, and likability were much higher than they expected. "Now, I go out of my way to talk to strangers," Sandstrom told me. "Even though I'm still an introvert."

If you'd still rather scrub toilets than start up a conversation, social psychologist Jolanda Jetten, a research professor at the University of Queensland, shows how we can benefit from social connection by simply belonging to a group, even when we're not having face-to-face contact with other group members. Her studies showed that group membership—such as supporting a professional sports team or advocacy group—regardless of the strength of individual ties within the group, or even physical proximity, improves well-being.[12] We can still feel like a community member, even when our ability to connect in person is impeded by a lockdown, illness, or remote location. Coming together for virtual or in-person religious services, recreational activities, social movements, or cultural events can create the bonding needed to quiet our separation distress alarms.

"We have all these devices that measure our steps," says Jetten. "Maybe we need to start measuring the social connections that people have and help them make plans on how to expand their social network."

TIPS FOR MAXIMIZING THE HEALTH BENEFITS OF SOCIAL CONNECTION

- PAY ATTENTION TO POTENTIAL CONNECTION: We can practice moving our attention out of our heads (and devices) and into our environments, paying attention to potential opportunities for connection.

- COUNT OUR "SOCIAL STEPS": Small acts add up. What baby steps can we take? Remember that even brief eye contact, smiles, and greetings impact our well-being.

- START EASY: What are the easiest steps to take? We can start with people who appear more receptive to connection to build confidence, or start in areas where we're most comfortable.

- ESTABLISH A PULL MECHANISM: Pull mechanisms draw people into talking to us. For example, when I walk with my friend's dog, people stop to comment on how cute he is. During the pandemic, we built a community library box in front of our home, so strangers constantly stop by to give and take books, making it easy to chat with them.

- RETHINK PRODUCTIVITY: We can move our intentions from being time-efficient to wellness-efficient by choosing to greet or chat with a stranger in the same way we'd choose to take the stairs to increase our steps. If possible, prioritize the human contact when choosing between self-checkout or a cashier, online shopping or in-person, texting or calling.

- **KEEP PRACTICING**: One of Sandstrom's studies showed that daily practice made people more confident and less fearful of rejection when starting conversations.[13]

- **INCREASE REMINDERS OF BELONGING**: We can increase our membership and affiliation with more groups, such as social movements, spiritual and support groups, teams, political parties, recreational groups, and communities of practice. Reminders of these affiliations, such as photos or symbols, can also tell our separation distress alarm that we're connected and safe.

- **CONNECTION TO PURPOSE**: We can anchor in our seeking and care systems to ground us through stormy times. What do we each care about? How does this bond us to the collective and strengthen it? What activities can we each pursue to connect us to this purpose? Is there a way to collaborate or share these efforts with others?

THE RELATIONSHIP MATTERS MOST

When a team researched the effectiveness of antidepressants in people experiencing a depressed episode, as expected, they found that those receiving the antidepressant did better on average than those taking the placebo.[14] But they also found that each prescribing psychiatrist had markedly different outcomes when offering the same intervention. Who offered the treatment impacted the participants' outcomes more than whether they received the active medication or placebo. A third of the psychiatrists even provided better outcomes with the placebo than a third of psychiatrists did with the active medication. The researchers concluded, "The clinician is not only the provider of treatment, but the means of treatment."

The same is true for psychotherapy. It's not the specific techniques of unique therapies that impact outcome, but the quality of the therapeutic relationship that matters most. It's true for so many other professions, too.

And yet so much of our education focuses on mastering knowledge, techniques, and concrete skills. I mentioned before how we chose a preschool with absolutely no focus on academics for our kids. We laughed that all the parents who threw their kids in this nonacademic school were academics themselves—psychiatrists, child psychologists, doctors, and professors. What the school did focus on was social and emotional development, which can be more important—and challenging—to develop. My children are older now, and with every parent-teacher meeting, I never focus on their academic skills. But I do ask a lot of questions about their social and emotional worlds at school. Are they showing kindness and connection to others? Are they capable of expressing their needs and participating in class? How are they showing up emotionally at school? Are there any challenges or conflicts I can support them with?

I supervise a lot of psychiatry residents in this same way. I see no need to endlessly quiz them on the content of our profession. That part is easy to learn. Instead, we focus on how we show up for our patients in the relationship. I hope to model and nurture the practice of kind attention, validation, curiosity, and compassion, toward both ourselves and our patients. We work to build comfort in not knowing and holding multiple perspectives, and in both being with a patient's pain and addressing conflict as an opportunity for growth. When we train as a therapist or mindfulness teacher, the most vital step in our education is to participate ourselves in the practices, whether getting our own therapy or attending mindfulness groups and retreats. We need to make these practices a lifestyle so we embody them from the inside out. It's not what we offer others, but how we offer it that matters most.

RELATIONSHIPS ARE MESSY

This social connection thing may all sound wonderful on paper, but when we get down to actually connecting with others, it often feels more stressful than going at it alone. For this reason, much of the fo-cus in psychotherapy is on how to improve our relationships.

I teach our psychiatry residents interpersonal therapy (IPT), a style of psychotherapy developed as a placebo condition for a medication trial in 1969, before we had scientific evidence that psychotherapy is effective. The biologically-oriented researchers at the time didn't yet understand how supportive counseling around a patient's relationships would have an impact on something as serious as a major depressive disorder.[15] But they found this "placebo" talk therapy that contained "no active ingredients" surprisingly effective.[16] Now, it's a first-line treat-ment for depression, with over 250 studies supporting its effective-ness in people with a number of physical and mental health conditions around the world.

IPT addresses our knowledge that depressive and other mental health episodes occur within interpersonal contexts of either unmet needs or disruptions in our relationships and social roles, such as con-flict, loss, and role transitions (like retiring or becoming a parent). Even desirable events and transitions can dysregulate us in the same way un-desired stressors do, because the uncertainty and changes in our roles are stressful.

In IPT, we explore effective ways to identify and feel our emo-tions, understanding them as signals that link to social threats or un-met rewards. We then learn to communicate these feelings and social needs to improve our relationships in the here and now.[17]

We can borrow some IPT strategies to help us explore our own interpersonal landscape, such as mapping out our *interpersonal inven-tory* to identify sources of potential support and conflict.[18] In the cen-ter circle below, right next to ME, we can jot down who is in our inner circle of intimacy, perhaps our partner, family, or best friends. In the next circle, we can add in the relationships that are of moderate intimacy, and then lower intimacy in the outer circle, such as other friends, colleagues, classmates, relatives, professional supports, reli-gious leaders, neighbors, and so on.

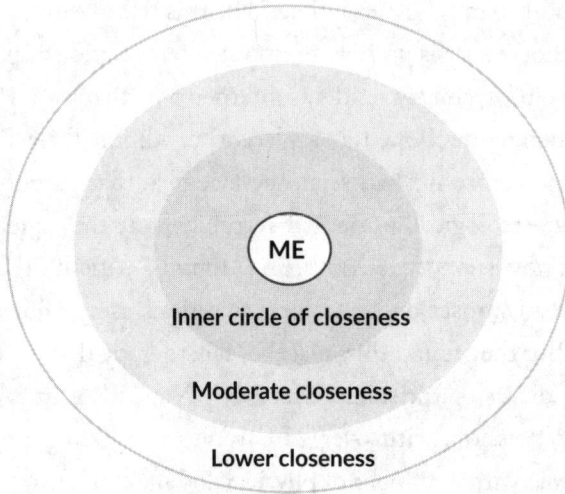

If we wish a relationship to be either closer or more boundaried, we can place an arrow from the person toward the place we'd like them to be in our circle. For example, if there's someone we hope to have more boundaries with, we may move the arrow from the inner circle to the outer. Or if we'd like to focus on improving the quality or quantity of contact with someone, we may place an arrow from an outer ring toward a closer one.

We can then consider each person in our inventory and reflect on:

1. WHAT do we like and not like about the relationship, thinking of examples for why?

2. HOW comfortable or capable are we in:
   - telling them how we feel, especially our vulnerable experiences?
   - asking for support?
   - talking about problems and conflicts?

3. HOW do we feel when we're with each person:
   - when things are going well?
   - when we're stressed or depleted?

- when we need support?
- when we're in conflict?

4. WHAT would we like to change in each relationship, reflecting on how we might feel if those things were different?

5. WHOM do we want to reconnect with more or deepen our connection to? Whom do we wish to have firmer boundaries with?
   - What steps can we take to attempt this?

6. WHAT changes in our own behaviors and assumptions could assist us in improving our current relationships?

When we run into conflicts or tension in our relationships, IPT teaches us to practice a *communication analysis*, where we try to bring the specific events of the entire interaction into our awareness. Dialectical behavior therapy (DBT) uses a similar strategy called a *behavioral chain analysis*. We move away from general statements filled with assumptions (for example, *"She got mad/rejected me"* or *"He always shuts down"*) and focus on the specifics of what really happened, exploring the actual words exchanged and behaviors observed, while reflecting on what was going on internally each step of the way. We can link our interpersonal behaviors with the specific emotions and level of activation that arose at the time.

For example, *He said, "You're late," and I noticed my body felt activated into shame as I assumed he was rejecting me. I tried to defend myself and said in an angry voice, "You're the one who never values my time." He appeared activated and angry then, too. He told me, "Why do you always have to turn everything into a fight?" I felt more shame and noticed myself shutting down into numbness and felt an urge to hide and avoid the discomfort, so I walked away.* This can be a challenging skill to begin with because we're often not used to tracking our internal experiences in such detail, but with practice, it becomes a well-trodden path.

Once we've brought to our awareness what happened both inside and outside of us, we can reflect on:

1. WHAT did we expect to happen in the interaction? We did we hope for?
   - How does this compare to what did happen in the interaction?

2. HOW much do we think the other person understood what we were trying to communicate?

3. WHAT do we think the other person's expectations and hopes were for the interaction?

4. WHAT are the short-term and long-term consequences of our behaviors?

5. WHAT might be more effective strategies to manage the situation in the future with what we now know?

We can then practice more helpful ways of communicating. We can begin by looking inward, learning to notice where we each are on the dial of activation, practicing regulation skills, and choosing a time to address the conflict when neither person is too activated or shut down so our prefrontal cortexes are online. We can observe what emotions and assumptions arise within us in the interaction and listen to what they're trying to signal about the situation. We can also evaluate whether these alarms are signaling true threats in the present, or false alarms from past learning or our negativity bias.

When we're ready to approach the other person, we can use *I statements* and watch out for blaming or shaming *you statements* (for example, "*You always get angry*"). If we notice we've regressed in this way to opposing teams, we can acknowledge the breakdown of communication and either take a time-out or work together to get back on the same team. Sometimes, it's as simple as saying, *"It feels like we're no longer on the same team right now,"* *"I'm noticing shame and blame are coming up between us,"* or *"I'm feeling we've moved out of connection, so can we take a pause to explore what's happening for both of us right now?"* In these moments, stepping out of the content of the conflict and into the process can be helpful to get us out of autopilot and to drive manually through a rocky section. When we're regulated enough to return to the conversation, we can explore and validate each other's feelings, needs, circumstances, and expectations.

Two strategies from DBT can help in these challenging moments. The first is to remember our dialects, that two (or more) opposing truths can exist at the same time. We can learn to hold multiple perspectives as equally valid: to both accept AND change, be flexible AND stable, nurturing AND challenging, and capable AND have limitations. For example, if we feel disappointed that someone canceled plans with us, we might acknowledge that it makes sense that they need the flexibility to cancel, as we accept their limitations and offer compassion, *and also* we can acknowledge our disappointment in the plans being changed and how it impacts us. If we really need the person to show up, we could offer compassion and accept their limitations *and also* communicate how much we need them and wonder if there's anything we could do to make it so they could still come. Notice how we say *and* instead of *but*. *But* infers that the second part of the statement is more important, while *and* implies that both realities are valid and true.

DBT and other types of therapy, like emotion-focused therapies, teach us to help each other co-regulate with validation. Remember how validation tells the brain that its alarms have been heard so it doesn't need to keep sounding? For example, if our friend tells us that he's canceling because his partner broke up with him out of the blue and he's been crying in bed for days, we could validate his experience in the following ways:

1. VALIDATE in the context of the present situation: "*It makes sense that this would be so painful as you two were planning a future together.*"

2. VALIDATE in the context of past experiences: "*It makes sense that this is especially painful as your last partner left in the exact same way.*"

3. VALIDATE with shared humanity: "*Ugh. Aren't breakups one of the most painful parts of life?*"

Emotion-focused family therapy (EFFT) teaches us to validate our children in at least three different ways, because it often takes the brain a while to get the message that the alarms are heard. For example, when one of my sons starts blaming me for things that don't feel like my fault, instead of paying attention to the content that's spewing out of his angry state and reacting defensively, I can observe the process of him feeling anger and get curious, perhaps responding, "*Hey love, there's a lot of anger here right now. Did something happen today to bring it on?*"

I could then practice validating all the reasons it makes sense he's angry, including both ones he's told me about and ones I'm guessing may also be at play. In EFFT, we learn to validate with *because* statements. For example, I could say, "*It makes so much sense you're angry because (1) you didn't get to go outside today at recess and lunch because it was pouring rain, and (2) you also had to sit in class all day doing subjects you don't like, and (3) your best friend is away, and I bet you miss him, and (4) you must be so tired and hungry after a long day of school. I imagine it's been a hard day!*"

Notice, instead of pointing out the invalid part—that I didn't think I did anything wrong to deserve this blame, amping him up more (and in full honesty, when they push my buttons hard, I struggle with falling into this unhelpful trap more often than I'd like to admit)—I acknowledge the valid part: he's angry and there's always a good reason why.

Sometimes, our internal experiences are valid because of the present situation, and sometimes, they're valid because of the past, but they're always valid. Our unskillful behaviors, though—like blaming your mom or beating up your brother when you've had a bad day at school—often aren't valid or helpful. DBT teaches us to only validate the valid parts while communicating boundaries on what behaviors are not okay. We can validate the anger and desire to act on it in unhelpful ways, but not the unhelpful action itself. For example, I could say, *"It makes sense that you're feeling so angry and wish you could beat up your brother or get mad at me to get some of that anger out. And also, hurting people isn't okay. I wonder how I can support you to be with this anger?"*

Once his anger alarm has been heard, he no longer needs to attack his authority figure to regain his agency. Instead, he settles, and we feel we're on the same team again. From this place, perhaps a bit later when he's back online, I can address the hurt this behavior caused me. For example, I might say, *"Hey, love, is this a good time to chat about what happened earlier? I know you had a really hard day and it makes so much sense you were really angry after school. And also, when you said those things to me, I felt really hurt. I want you to know the impact it had on me so we can work together to find ways to stay on the same team in these moments, because our relationship really matters to me. What do you think would be helpful for these hard moments next time so we can support you in your anger without pushing me away?"*

Then we can work collaboratively, maintaining his sense of agency, to problem-solve for the future. This approach also leads with bonding, reminding him that we're on the same team and I'm bringing it up because our relationship matters to me and I love him. I also add in the boundary that it's not okay for his behaviors to hurt me. Healthy boundaries allow me to stay on his team, because my capacity to offer him compassion requires them. The boundaries also help him feel less anxious, because they create more containment and certainty, so he consistently knows what behavior is okay and not okay. We can add to that feeling of containment by creating a plan together of how we could both try to respond next time to support him best in challenging moments. In this way, we offer the ABCs to calm his alarm systems.

Despite all this reflecting, problem-solving, and planning, there will still be many future times when we'll get triggered into anger, just like everyone else, deactivating our prefrontal cortex, so we act out in unhelpful ways. But because we've addressed these hard moments consistently with co-regulation before, we learn to self-regulate with ease. Last night, I overheard my boys fighting and it got physical. Before I could even get to them, I heard one son take space in his room for a moment, then come back, be accountable for his actions, and apologize to his brother. Then they moved on quickly, without needing my support, and were back on the same team.

You can see how this approach differs from punishment, which tends to dysregulate us further. If I were to respond immediately with, *"You can't talk to me that way. You have no respect. You're grounded,"* I would take away his agency and push us onto different teams. He would likely fight back against my power play, getting even more angry and dysregulated. Then the disconnect might trigger his separation distress alarm, too. If my punishments were inconsistent, so he never knew how I'd respond, I'd also trigger his fear alarm because of the lack of containment and predictability. This is *co-dysregulation.*

In all honesty, I have my moments where I've had a rough day or have low resources and go this route. I may have canceled Christmas one year, only to take it back an hour later. I've also taken away screens for the rest of eternity, which, you can probably guess, didn't last long either, although those minutes of dysregulation felt like forever. It rarely lands well. In these heated moments, we need to take our own time-out to get back into balance before we can help co-regulate anyone else and offer a skillful repair.

As we practice this more often, and within the same relationship, we can learn to notice tension earlier, before it erupts into problems, just like practicing kind attention to our own experiences helps us catch challenges while they're still small. For example, my partner and I frequently focus our kind attention skills on each other, commenting that the other seems a bit activated (or in my case, deactivated), and asking if there's anything we'd like to talk about or get support for. Sometimes, my partner is validly annoyed by my annoying actions—I have many, just like everyone else—and I'm able to understand my impact on her, validate it, and repair before it grows into a bigger problem. Sometimes, she's worried about outside things and needs my support. And sometimes, it's a false alarm, with me projecting my past onto her. We can be careful that we don't compulsively overdo it, so that the checking in itself becomes irritating, something I've struggled with because of my jumpy separation alarm in past stressful seasons of life.

OUR PAST HASN'T PASSED

Focusing on the impacts of our relationships in our present environment doesn't negate that our past relationships also impact how we meet today's social challenges. How we show up today in relationships depends on how others have shown up for us in the past, especially when we're under stress and our threat alarms are more sensitive.

Freud is famous for recognizing that we all have an unconscious. He likened the mind to an iceberg, where only the tip that we see above the water is conscious. The vast majority of the mind's functions that affect how we think, feel, and behave are submerged, operating implicitly, outside of our awareness.

Therapists talk of *projection* to describe the unconscious process of transferring our past learning about the world—and particularly the people in it—onto the person standing in front of us. If we've learned that others have fragile, abusive, inconsistent, or dishonest parts from past relationships, then we will project this pattern of perceiving others onto our present relationships, especially if they possess something that fits our projection and sets off our alarm.

My training psychoanalyst once told me, "We project onto reality," meaning that the person we project onto often shares something with the source of our past learning. For example, when people possess a stiff, unanimated face, my historical alarm tells me that they may reject me. This happens unconsciously, usually with a subtle shame alarm. I might not even be aware that my mind's shooting me *You're not enough* or *You're going to be rejected* warnings. Until I become mindful of my activation and get curious, I'll likely instinctively believe I'm in danger of rejection and armor up or hide.

Even though I've implicitly learned that this facial expression is associated with people in the past rejecting me, it's not the facial expression itself that does the rejecting. In fact, many people show these expressions when they're anxious or uncomfortable, perhaps when they're afraid of being rejected themselves. If I listen to my alarm and instinctively assume this person in front of me is threatening when they're actually socially anxious, I may act in ways that lead to the rejection we both fear.

We can learn to notice when we're experiencing an alarm from implicit memory by observing our body for signs of getting activated or shut down. First, we may need to seek safety and soothe our nervous systems before we have the capacity to evaluate the alarm with perspective. Then we can assess if it's pushing us toward a helpful response in the present. When we bring such awareness to our implicit alarms, we create the space to choose the most useful responses, rather than habitually abide by their demands in autopilot.

We can also explore the history of our alarms to understand that they make sense because of our past, even when they are firing too often in our present. In this way, we can validate them as helpful adaptations rather than a sign that we're malfunctioning.

Patrisse Cullors, a cofounder of Black Lives Matter, shows us how these projections impact our teams:

There's a lot of trauma that we project on each other. And in that trauma projection, we become each other's enemies, truly. And we fall short of being able to make assessments that are not grounded in our trauma . . . Because oftentimes what I see is, we are all in it, but we're not all in it together.[19]

Because our historical alarms can make us believe that the people in front of us right now are past perpetrators of harm, it's challenging to stay on the same team when we're all projecting at the same time, as Cullors describes, turning our communications into a mosaic of false assumptions.

We see this so often in romantic relationships, too. We love and want the best for each other and our relationship, but then we suddenly get triggered into a historical alarm and see our partner as the people who've hurt us most in the past. Then we communicate with them from this projection, triggering them, too, so we both become less capable of truly seeing and relating to each other from the same team.

We also might lack the capacity to be curious because of low internal or external resources at the time, outside of the interpersonal conflict. When our world is on fire, and we're in crisis mode, can't make rent, or we're sick, depressed, or stressed, our nervous systems move into their stress responses to survive. Again, we lose access to our upstairs brain that allows us to pause, evaluate whether our projections and alarms are accurate to the present situation, and tease out what information is useful to drive the bus in the right direction. That's why when Cullors observes that her group is no longer on the same team, she asks, "What does it take to resource all of us, so that we can be in this together?"

When we're all grating on each other—assuming that our loved ones or colleagues are jerks or about to abandon us—we can ask ourselves, *What internal and external resources do we all need right now to have the capacity to have compassion and curiosity for exploring what's really going on inside us?* Sometimes, it's simply a break or snack.

Often, it's healthier boundaries, when possible. When we're lacking boundaries with others, we may quickly become overwhelmed and lose our capacity to be generous and curious in our assumptions. We also can't settle into our slower upstairs brain to notice that so much of our conflict is projections from our past relationships.

Cullors suggests we anchor in our values and commitments to help us drive in the direction we want, even when our inner passengers from the past are heckling up a riot. When I trained as a Daring Way facilitator with Brené Brown's team, they had us choose two core values that would act as our personal compass in these confusing and activating moments. We then wrote these two values on our name tags. As we worked together, whenever we became overwhelmed by our internal hecklers, they instructed us to look down at our name tag and use our values to steer us in the right direction.

FEELING IT TO HEAL IT

While we often get frustrated when we find ourselves triggered by historical alarms or projecting our pasts onto people in the present, we can remember that these moments of feeling our past hurts are the best path to healing them. We need to reexperience our split-off emotional states and their implicit relational learning to make them conscious and integrate them back into our awareness. Because so many of our past hurts feel intolerable, especially when they occurred in childhood at a time when we often didn't have the internal and external resources to hold the pain like we do now, we fragment them off from our awareness and bury them deep in our unconscious, where they remain dormant until a similar situation detonates them unexpectedly at the least convenient times. Then they hijack our bus because we haven't had practice in allowing them to sit peacefully in the passenger seat.

By bringing these states back into awareness, allowing them to sit in plain view on the bus with us, we can learn that we now have more internal and external resources to hold them, without pushing them back into hiding. We heal by integrating all our parts back into balance so that no one part hides in the trunk or grabs the steering wheel.

Psychoanalysis and its hip younger sister, psychodynamic therapy, identify *object relations*—with *object* being the peculiar word its founders chose to describe people—to explain how we implicitly assume new relationships will act like the more threatening or frustrating relationships of our past, especially those from our family of origin, since they taught us early on what behaviors to expect from others.

We project our past relationship dynamics between two people, not simply the individual traits of one part of the pair. For example, we aren't insecurely attached people, but we can have insecurely attached relationships. I can feel very securely attached with people who relate to me in secure ways. I can also feel anxious in relation to someone important to me who's relating to me in avoidant ways. It's a play with two parts: we implicitly learn that there's a perpetrator and victim, an inattentive caregiver and unseen child, a dependent underfunctioner and a caregiving overfunctioner. We not only project expected traits onto someone, but we also identify with the counter role, because we've internalized the relationship dynamic between the pair.

I've internalized from my past a pattern of feeling unseen and fearing abandonment in relationships while expecting others to be either inattentive or unreliable, even when the present people in my life are consistently present for me. This implicit learning from the past has kept me safe: in some situations, I can set low expectations and prepare for others to act in a way that mimics my past relationships, so I'm not disappointed when my needs can't be met with new people. But it can also become a self-fulfilling prophecy: at times, I can feel so concerned about losing my connection to others that I try too hard to keep them around. This can feel intrusive, so others may pull away and re-create my past relational pattern. We call this an *enactment*, when our historical alarms or projections from the past sometimes make us act in ways that push our present relationships to behave just like those of our past.

And then it gets even trickier, because we can also flip into playing the opposite role of an internalized relationship, projecting the other side of the relational pattern onto others. So, in other situations, I inhabit the role of seeming absent or unreliable to others and they inhabit the role of feeling unseen or neglected. Between the two roles, this one feels more empowering because it's less dependent on anyone else, so I rest here when I'm really stressed and can't bear the pain of my needs for connection being unmet. At the same time, others can be put off by my apathy and disengage with me, which is the opposite outcome to securing the connection I so deeply desire.

Complicating it even further, we've taken in many different relationship dynamics from the many important people of our past who shaped our assumptions of what to expect from others. I've also internalized a dominant role interacting with a submissive one. So, when others express a hint of dominance or anger, I often feel a need to passively submit, fawn, or shut down, even when they're communicating healthy expressions of anger. At other times, though, when I'm really pushed into my defensive mode, my fight response may lead me to play the opposite side as the dominant part. This is what my loved ones call my "cool and calculated" flavor of anger, with its capacity to tear a strip out of someone while still smiling, leaving the other speechless and submissive.

When you internalize a relationship dynamic, you don't get to inhabit only one role of it. And while playing the opposite part of our past may feel unwelcome, it's still adaptive in extreme situations. This role comes out when I need to fight the system for a patient to receive their disability insurance or appropriate treatment. My patients frequently come to their appointment in disbelief, reporting that their caseworker is now scared of me and will agree to their need for coverage, wondering how the gentle trauma therapist they know so well in session could possibly have such a frightening effect on their gatekeeper to services.

Often when I talk about these parts of myself openly, people are surprised that I'm revealing such socially undesirable traits. But psychological health is not eliminating these unattractive parts of our-selves. It's learning to acknowledge that we all have adapted to our environments by internalizing many relational dynamics to survive. We learn to accept them all as a part of us.

We often assume that we have a static personality that doesn't change. But we react to different situations with a large variety of states, each with its own pattern of thinking, feeling, and behaving, based on what past implicit memories and alarms the unique situation triggers in us.

Internal Family Systems therapy (IFS) identifies these different states as adaptive versions of our younger selves that have been split off from our *going on with normal life* adult self.[20] When we've been exposed to adversity, it can be adaptive to disown our unmet needs and socially unacceptable feelings and urges. We may perceive these parts as bad, while trying to preserve the rest of us as all good. But these experiences still exist within us in split-off parts.

"Living through the battlefield of our outside world has created a minefield within me," one of my mindfulness participants told our group, as he described how a lifetime of overriding these painful experiences left them fragmented off from his *going on with normal life* self and ready to detonate at unexpected times. Sometimes, our split-off parts take over and drive our behaviors. They fully inhabit us, and we are unable to see them as just parts of a much bigger whole.

When a past partner and I were in our *going on with normal life* self-state, and almost all our other ones, too, we were full of empathy and seemingly perfectly matched in every way. Except for one. "Our conscious selves love each other," I told her toward the end of our relationship. "But our unconscious parts are at war."

When we fought, our unique interpersonal dance triggered implicit relational patterns that we both didn't usually inhabit with others. It was only one of our many relational parts that clashed. Unfortunately, it was the pattern that we both jumped into when extremely hurt, and the more conflict it created, the more hurt we became, leaving us dys-regulating in these feuding parts too often.

Our couples therapist, trained in IFS, had us identify these parts as inhabiting our *adaptive child modes* rather than being bad. She could see us start a session joyfully driving the bus on the same team. But when hurt came up, we quickly had a costume change into our adaptive child modes of armoring up or shutting down. We learned to name these modes when they arose and take mindful pauses when we needed time to pull them away from the steering wheel. We developed a lot of understanding and compassion for these parts in ourselves and each other, validating where they came from by linking them to how each of us adapted to our past hurts in old relationships.

But still, we eventually chose to break up. We didn't like how often we were pushed into these painful parts of ourselves, despite learning how to work with them. As I continued to date, I realized that I delighted in, shared values with, and got along with many people. However, it wasn't until I spent enough time in each relationship, particularly in hard times and conflict, that I could see the compatibility of our inner workings.

When I met my current partner, I immediately fell for her. While she ticked every box, with so many gorgeous qualities to admire, I also loved the person I was when with her, all the time, even when stressed into my adaptive states. While we're optimistic about our future, it takes time to fully trust that it will last, because we need to weather many storms together to prove we can stay curious, compassionate, and on the same team when all our stressed-out parts decide to pop in and say hello from the depths of our unconsciouses.

As in every intimate relationship, all these parts make cameos, and some play recurrent roles. But as we both meet each other's hurt passengers with care, showing us that they aren't so scary after all, we get the chance to see and hold all of their rowdiness in a safe and loving environment. In this process of reactivating these past hurts and then having them received in this way, we're healing them. The key is to go to where the love is, where we can learn that others can also be sources of safety, tenderness, and attunement.

It's never too late to internalize healthy relationships into our psyche. One of the participants of a therapy group I facilitate shared with us that all the unruly passengers of shame, anxiety, scarcity, and trauma on her internal bus were hollering at her to turn the bus around as she tried to steer it toward an important goal. "But then I pictured all of you on the bus, too. Every one of you, accepting me and offering support and compassion," she said. "And the scary passengers were still there, but all of you were there, too, all on the bus with them, cheering me on to keep steering it forward. You outnumbered them."

HOW POWER IMPACTS RELATIONSHIPS

I sought out my current therapist for her expertise in anti-oppression and justice-oriented therapy. Her clinic focuses on counseling equity-deserving populations, accepting me as a client because of my queerness. But when we had our first session, I told her that it's my position of so much unearned social power and privilege that brought me to therapy. I was aware of my positionality as a healthy white settler and physician living in Canada, but I felt so much shame and guilt for the inequities that I benefit from that I became too distressed to do anything useful about it. Just like we split off our hurt parts, I unconsciously disowned these undesired parts that held power and privilege.

When we reflect on our positions of intersectionality—that is, the complex and cumulative ways in which many forms of marginalization, such a racism, sexism, and classism, intersect—we see that power is multidimensional and unbalanced in a variety of ways. We can hold positions of power in some areas and not others. Because our mirror neurons allow us to feel what others in our collective are facing—as long as stress hasn't shut us down into the freeze state of indifference—it's common to feel guilt and shame when we acknowledge that our unevenly distributed positions of power and privilege come from the inequities of others losing theirs. It's so much more comfortable to focus on the areas where we don't hold power and privilege, such as my identity as a queer woman. When, in fact, in the game of life, the cards have always been unfairly stacked in my favor.

My therapist pointed out how I related to this power I held as all bad, trying to deny or get rid of it. "Power itself isn't bad," she told me. "It's what we do with it. You can use your power to dominate over others, or you can use it to empower them. Just like you've learned to hold all your vulnerable parts tenderly, can you learn to hold your power without judgment, too, so you don't need to disown it?" She helped me befriend my power and privilege so that I could acknowledge these dynamics, exploring how I can best use my power to empower others and transform our systems into ones that are more equitable for everyone.

Sociologist Manuel Castells, a professor at the Universitat Oberta de Catalunya, described how the nature of power in our social world is in connecting people and groups through networks. We can either share our power by linking others to social networks, or we can hoard power by excluding others with gatekeeping and hierarchies.

Even in groups fighting against oppression, when our societies are rooted in supremacy and subordination, we, too, often find ourselves reproducing these internalized dynamics with one another, though we exercise superiority in different ways. In her book, *Burnout: The Emotional Experience of Political Defeat*, historian Hannah Proctor reminds us that many anti-oppression movements tried to work together in nonhierarchical ways only to find it really, really hard. She references the Red Therapy collective, who struggled to put their nonhierarchical theory into practice. "We couldn't somehow will ourselves liberated and wake up the next morning feeling wonderfully collective, non-jealous, confident, non-competitive, etc. We couldn't suddenly change the patterns of a lifetime which we had been forced to conform to in this society," she wrote.

While social movements explicitly understand how members need to relate to one another to create a healthy society—with unity, equity, compassion, and the celebration of diversity—we're still implicitly programmed from a lifetime of living in a hierarchical culture of dominance, division, and disposability. And we can be hard on ourselves and each other when our unconscious selves take the wheel, enacting old dynamics that drive us away from our ideals.

In this way, building diverse, intergenerational movements always creates conflict, explain organizers Kelly Hayes and Mariame Kaba in *Let This Radicalize You: Organizing and the Revolution of Reciprocal Care*. "But the desire to shrink groups down to spaces of easy agreement is not conducive to movement building," they teach.[21] Today's culture of zero tolerance for mistakes deprives us of learning from constructive feedback and repair within relationships, they warn. Instead, they ask, can we support each other's growth with compassion and curiosity, so we can come together to build movements large enough to fight the forces that, left unchecked, will destroy us all?

We might find these destructive dynamics enacted when we demand perfect language, knowledge, and behavior from each other. We are diverse people who are constantly shaped by the specific cultures we inhabit. We also each have different access to education and social and psychological resources. Group facilitator Priya Parker teaches in *The Art of Gathering* that when we don't explicitly share social norms, people from diverse backgrounds can feel anxious because they don't know how they should act to belong. I'm terrified to put this book out there because I know my unique conditioning likely won't land well with so many others around the world. I have no idea what all my readers' social norms are, and I could never please everyone.

Yes, language and behavior matter, and we must all try our best to learn from others to ensure our actions are as safe and inclusive as possible. And also, harm is inevitable, especially when we've all been socialized in such different ways. It's easy to fall into the superiority of shunning people when they don't have the same education and cultural upbringings in specific areas as we do. When we push people away for making mistakes, we exclude them from learning and repairing the wounds, dividing and weakening our collective even more.

While we need healthy boundaries about what behavior is not okay to protect our collective from harm, it's also through contact and care that our divisions heal, through showing up and allowing each other to see our vulnerabilities underneath all our ugly cloaks of conditioning. We need to create a culture of belonging, where we acknowledge the uncomfortable mess of being human in a dysregulated world and try to grow together, not one that depends on a narrow definition of perfection or fantasies of good and evil to fit in.

In *We Will Not Cancel Us,* movement mediator adrienne maree brown reminds us that cancel and call-out culture originated as a way for marginalized people to stop harm and abuse from those who hold power over them, not "to shame and humiliate people in the wake of misunderstandings, contradictions, conflicts, and mistakes." When we punish and subordinate each other, we weaken our movements, she explains.

"If this kind of call outs sweeping through online organizing space and spilling into real-life formations actually stopped harm, resolved conflict, ended supremacy, and transformed people, I'd be a gung-ho call-out machine! I love functional tools," brown says. But instead, people move apart, leave movements, or double down and return with even more egregious acts of flagrant harm, she argues. Instead, we need to move our efforts toward having hard conversations. We can strive not for perfection or the pleasure of revenge, but for the healing of moving through the process of naming what caused harm, understanding what happened and what is needed for repair, and then offering accountability and apologies or reparations, while committing to paths of unlearning these harmful belief systems and behaviors.

"We need the people within our movements, all socialized into and by unjust systems, to be on liberation paths," brown continues. "Not already free, but practicing freedom every day. Not already beyond harm, but accountable for doing our individual and internal work to end harm and engage in generative conflict, which includes actively working to gain awareness of the ways we can and have harmed each other . . . and where we can end cycles of harm. I want our movements to feel like a vibrant, accountable space where causing harm does not mean you are excluded immediately and eternally from healing, justice, community, or belonging."

We're often derailed in our efforts to repair by confusing conflict with abuse. In abuse, there is a misuse of power, with the person exhibiting both a harmful behavior and power over the other, as we explored in Chapter Five. In conflict, there isn't this misuse of power, although there still may be a power struggle, since all human relationships have power dynamics. When we overstate harm by mislabeling conflict as abuse, we then become the party misusing power, by shunning members of our collective instead of healing the fracture with a skillful repair, explains activist Sarah Schulman in *Conflict Is Not Abuse: Overstating Harm, Community Responsibility, and the Duty of Repair.*

Schulman diagnoses the unjustified escalation of conflict into abuse as a symptom of both poles in the dynamics of dominance: the entitlement of supremacy and the trauma of subordination. First, this happens frequently with those in positions of dominance who feel entitled to emotional comfort and control, while refusing to admit mistakes or hear information they don't like. These people are safe to express their complaints (and they expect them to be addressed), unlike those in marginalized positions, who are often harmed by the police, courts, and community when they sound the alarm.

When someone in a subordinated position challenges the person in a position of dominance's superior self-concept with the accurate feedback that their behavior caused harm, those in dominant positions often feel discomfort and equate the discomfort with abuse, even though they are the ones exerting power over the other and causing harm. They may feel hurt, but they aren't being harmed and subordinated. They're uncomfortable and don't have the skills or motivation to stay with the emotional alarm of guilt long enough to be accountable and address the problem.

Sometimes, the person who is in a position of dominance inaccurately complains of abuse when the person being subordinated resists their power over them. For example, those who perpetrate abuse often use the power of the police, public opinion, or legal action to further control the people they abuse, accusing the subordinated party of "abuse" (or defamation) when they're only attempting to resist it, Schulman explains.

This, too, happens at a group and systems level, when those who resist oppression are seen as the offenders and punished for their attempts to free themselves from subordination, as with the recent backlash against diversity, equity, and inclusivity initiatives. At the United Nation's headquarters during the Commission on the Status of Women in 2025, many delegates from around the world warned of the growing "anti-rights movements" that undermine our long-standing consensus on universal human rights. A UN report published ahead of the meeting showed that a quarter of governments worldwide reported a regression in women's rights in 2024.[22]

In a panel addressing this backlash, Laura Nyirinkindi, the chair of the UN Working Group on discrimination against women and girls, explained how recognizing the reality of our intersectional identities is not inherently divisive, but rather an affront to our entrenched dynamics of domination and subordination. It's uncomfortable to face the reality that one's success is a result of unfairly hoarded privileges and power and not the "merit" of our fantasies, and even more uncomfortable to face policies that offer others the same safety and opportunities that have previously been reserved only for one's own dominant group. But it's not abuse. "Recognizing our intersectionality holds the power to identify and challenge systemic inequities and advocate for justice," Nyirinkindi said, while maintaining our universal human rights and common humanity.

On the other pole of the dynamic, we can mistake conflict for abuse when we have unhealed trauma from being subordinated and harmed in our pasts. We may unconsciously project our trauma dynamics onto the conflict, confusing it with abuse, when there is no current misuse of power and harm in the present relationship. Or we may feel incapable of holding uncomfortable emotions—especially when guilt quickly shifts into intense shame waves, as we see so often as a past adaptation to trauma—so constructive feedback feels threatening.

Sometimes, we've been conditioned to believe that only those who experience abuse will receive support, so we unconsciously inflate the harm as the only way we know to seek care. This is particularly true when we're living in righteous or punitive cultures that reduce people to only good/bad or abuser/victim statuses. But when we overuse the rhetoric of abuse and harm, Schulman explains, we desensitize our communities' alarms when it really does happen, threatening the safety of the huge number of people experiencing true abuse, who already struggle with being heard and helped.

In situations where we escalate conflict into the rhetoric of abuse, we might "assert boundaries" to shun the person or "hold them accountable" to take revenge. These approaches only regress us into using the oppressor's tools of dominating over, dividing, and disposing of others. Such attempts to prevent harm create more harm. Asserting boundaries and natural consequences are essential in healthy relationships in conflict. But boundaries need terms for repair, Shulman teaches. We might need someone to be accountable, sober, or attend therapy for a specific time period before we reengage with them. These terms may never be met, "But at least there is always a possibility of repair," Schulman explains. "Refusing to speak to someone without terms for repair is a strange, [regressed] act of destruction in which nothing can be won." She continues, "By refusing to talk without terms, a person is refusing to learn about themselves and thereby refusing to have a better life. It hurts everyone around them by dividing communities and inhibiting learning."

Of note, we need to remember that these strategies are suggested for people in situations of conflict, not abuse, which require a different approach, as we explored in Chapter Four. In these situations, stopping the harm and misuse of power is the priority, without the person being harmed holding the additional burden of educating the person who caused harm.

We often aren't even aware that we're causing more harm instead of stopping it. Because conflict is stressful, it pushes us into emotional states of fight, flight, or freeze, where we're prone to thinking traps, such as seeing the person associated with the anger, guilt, or shame that arises within us as all bad. Because we *feel* bad, we assume they must *be* bad since the interaction with them brought on these feelings. We're especially vulnerable to confusing conflict with abuse when we don't have the emotional and social skills or resources to cope with and make sense of the conflict.

"Unfortunately, it is the distorted social norm to see the wish to repair as an assault," Shulman explains. "The real question is: Why would a person rather have an enemy than a conversation?" Sometimes, we're more comfortable believing that the other is all bad than holding the complexities that our environments have conditioned us all to have different healthy and unhealthy parts that rub up against each other all the time. However, this withholding produces anxiety, Shulman adds, while accountability creates relief.

"Without conversation, it is the person with the most limitations who is in control. The desirable goal for all of us is not to restrict those who can, but to bring more communication skills to those who can't. Refusal through email, texting, and other technologies keeps the person who doesn't know how to problem-solve from learning how. It keeps them imprisoned in their own imagined negative fears about the other, and their fantasies of their own potential humiliation or demise if they were to talk to the other person and thereby understand what the other person is thinking and feeling," she argues.

When conflicts arise, we can practice wading into the discomfort by reflecting on the following questions:

1. HOW safe are you right now in your environment? What do you need to seek safety?

2. WHAT state of emotional activation are you in? Do you need time or space to return to balance before you can act from your most skillful self?

3. WHAT emotions are you experiencing? Are they primary emotions connected to the situation (for example, guilt for causing harm or shame when the current setting is punitive and rejecting) or secondary emotions confusing the situation (for example, we switched our guilt into shame, where we assume we're being rejected even when the situation is psychologically safe; or anger, when we blame others for our uncomfortable feelings, even when we caused the harm)?

4. ARE these true alarms alerting you to social danger right now or false alarms from the past? If historical, acknowledge and care for this pain first so you can approach the current conflict from a place of clarity.

5. ARE power over dynamics at play between parties right now? Are you unsafe from the abusive power imbalance in the relationship, or are you uncomfortable from the emotions triggered from the conflict? In what way? If there is a power over dynamic involved, is this at an individual, group, or systemic level?

6. ARE you on the same team right now? What might you need to return to the same team?

7. ARE your actions escalating or repairing the situation?

8. WHAT can you learn from this, and in what ways can you grow for next time?

ORGANIZING OUR COLLECTIVE

Whereas Charles Darwin popularized the concept of "survival of the fittest," evolutionary biologist Theodosius Dobzhansky argued that "the fittest may also be the gentlest, because survival often requires mutual help and cooperation."

Gustave Le Bon, a French social psychologist in the late 1800s, coined the term *group mind* to describe how individuals in groups regress into unhealthy behaviors, as each member takes less responsibility for their actions and feels their transgressions will go unnoticed.[23] At the same time, he observed how groups can enhance individual behavior, too, but only when there's organization, clear goals, and a common purpose.

Members of our social systems stay regulated and united when our subcortical alarms are calmed by the ABCs of agency, bonding, and containment. When a group begins to dysregulate, just as when individuals do, we can work to improve their sense of agency (by ensuring a sense of autonomy, equity, and justice), bonding (by connecting in safe and supportive cultures), and containment (by keeping them safe and offering consistent and clear boundaries and expectations).

Facilitator Priya Parker explains that while removing governance and regulations is tempting, renouncing leadership doesn't eradicate power imbalances in groups. Nor does it improve our freedom. It only leaves the power up for grabs for the least healthy members to swoop in, and they often use it in a dominating instead of empowering way. We don't want our groups to be at the mercy of unelected members who hoard power and privileges while dividing and harming others.

The kind of freedom we need most right now is not the freedom to harm—to dominate over, incite divisions, or destroy the people and ecosystems that we depend on to survive. We need the freedom from harm. And the freedom to live to our fullest potential so we can cultivate our diverse strengths to best support the health of our collective. For this reason, Parker recommends that we govern social systems with generous leadership to promote equity and empower members (agency), connect them (bonding), and protect each person from harm (containment).

Protection is largely preloaded explicitly in how we set up our social norms, Parker teaches. This clear and agreed upon set of boundaries and expectations anchors us to common processes when the storms hit. For example, if we all learn a process for repair when future conflicts and missteps inevitably arise, the storm doesn't feel so scary and uncertain.

In *Fumbling towards Repair*, community accountability facilitators Mariame Kaba and Shira Hassan explain that we can't "hold people accountable." People can only "take accountability," accepting responsibility for their own harmful actions. Blaming and shaming each other in conflicts are symptoms of regressing into the dynamics of domination, division, and disposibility, which only dysregulate us further, making us less capable of taking accountability. Instead, we can work to create the conditions of safety and support required for each of us to practice accountability for the parts we contributed to in each situation. We want to feel safe enough to listen to our guilt alarms that tell us our *behaviors* are problematic, so we can change them, not be shamed or blamed into believing *we* are bad, pushing us to deny and deflect responsibility.

Again, a prerequisite for this work is healthy boundaries to enforce what behaviors are not okay, especially when the person causing harm has not stopped the behavior. We can only extend compassion when boundaries prevent ongoing harm. But these boundaries need conditions for repair built into the contract.

Ruptures are inevitable, no matter how well our relationships and groups function. But ruptures themselves don't cause dysfunction in our relationships and systems; it's our inability to repair the disruption. Remember how I introduced the anxiety equation earlier? Anxiety is a function of our perception of the threat in comparison to our ability to cope with it. If we can build our capacity to repair our relationships, then our emotional alarms don't need to scream so loudly when conflict and harm inevitably occur.

Because I spent so much of my early life in shame waves, terrified of causing harm, learning that there's a path to repair my future mistakes alleviated my anxiety in a way that trying to prevent it never could. If we have a way to move through conflict, we no longer need to deflect and deny it, nor shame and blame others in attempts to feel better. As Maya Angelou advised, "Do the best you can until you know better, then when you know better, do better."

Whenever I find myself marinating in waves of guilt and shame over the inevitable missteps of being human, I turn to the work of artist and activist Alok (ALOK) Vaid-Menon for support.

"Being alive is about messing up gloriously," ALOK offers.[24] "What we do then is say, 'I'm sorry, I'm learning. It won't happen again.' And then if it happens again, we say, 'I'm sorry, I'm going to try even harder.' And that's what love is for me: trying harder for each other."

PRACTICING ACCOUNTABILITY

1. LISTEN DEEPLY WITH CURIOSITY TO UNDERSTAND THE IMPACT OF OUR ACTIONS ON OTHERS. Practice attending to the feedback with compassion and care toward both ourselves and the people we've hurt or harmed to stay in balance and out of defensiveness.

2. ACCEPT AND ACKNOWLEDGE THE IMPACT OF OUR ACTIONS (WITHOUT MINIMIZING THEM WITH EXCUSES OF GOOD INTENTIONS). As Ta-Nehisi Coates teaches in Between the World and Me, "'Good intention' is a hall pass through history," used to bypass accountability.

3. MAKE AMENDS WITH DIRECT APOLOGIES OR REPARATIONS TO THE PEOPLE WHOM WE'VE IMPACTED.

4. TAKE STEPS TO LEARN FROM THE EXPERIENCE TO CHANGE OUR BEHAVIORS IN THE FUTURE, SO WE DON'T HARM IN THE SAME WAY AGAIN.

5. IF THE HARM OCCURS AGAIN, WE MUST TRY EVEN HARDER, ESPECIALLY BEING CURIOUS TO WHAT LEARNING OR PRACTICES WE MISSED THE FIRST TIME.

In this way, I would like to be in relationship with any harmful impact this book causes, in particular, to those who hold less power and privilege than me, so I can acknowledge, learn, repair, and try my hardest to prevent it from occurring again.[25]

More than ever, we need a world where we can celebrate our capacity to see where we've gone wrong and then pivot toward a healthier path. It's never too late to acknowledge our mistakes and change, while extending each other compassion and opportunities to stay connected while we learn and grow. The resuscitation of our world depends on it.

EMERGING INTO BOUNDLESS POSSIBILITIES

In my mindfulness training, we learned of the centuries-old Japanese art form of *kintsukuroi* ("golden repair"). When pottery breaks, artists mend the cracks with a lacquer dusted with gold, silver, or platinum, shaping it into something more beautiful than its original form. When we invest in the process of rupture and repair, we, too, can transform our relationships into unions that are stronger than before.

As the world feels more broken than ever, we can still come back together to transform our fractured pieces into a new world that's brighter than the ones we've known. The pandemic crushed our fantasies that we could go at it alone, as we lost our health and stability when starved of each other. But, sometimes, we need the pieces shattered at our feet to see how poorly built our structures have been all along.

They say that the wrong people will find you in peace and leave you in pieces, but the right ones will find you in pieces and leave you in peace. I'm a believer in happy endings, in love prevailing for each other and for this world. As I cuddle on the couch with my partner, relishing in the remoteness of our island cabin, I notice that my hyperactive attachment alarm hasn't rung since I met her, despite isolating in the depths of my writing cave for months.

"You're my Rat Park," I tell her, squeezing her hand.

While she probably wishes she'd fallen for a poet, not a science geek, she understands me like no other. "I love you, too," she responds. And I know she's glued the many cracks of my well-used heart back together with gold.

All systems eventually come back into balance, even when they're forced to function in new ways. Western literature confined many of our imaginations to the dramatic arc of the Hero's Journey, a linear story with a crisis, climax, and resolution. It's how we often view resilience: the ability to bounce back to our former state in the face of stress.

But resilience can emerge in much more stunning and transformative ways. Instability generates new possibilities, just as plowing the soil creates the fertile ground for growth. When a system hits critical points of instability, wildly different adaptations can emerge out of the chaos of the old model's collapse.

Just like nature's movements take on many forms, our social movements aren't confined to the linear wave of the narrative arc. Our heroic revolutions can spiral, converge, meander, branch, bubble, or explode into a mosaic of unpredictable possibilities. While changes in our personal perspectives, values, actions, and relationships may feel insignificant in comparison to the gravity of our problems, small transformations in any one part or connection in our entangled system can change it in leaps and bursts.

New possibilities emerge when everyday people inspire those around them. A new connection can branch into a network of culture change; a viral moment can explode into a worldwide movement. Healthier ways of relating to each other and this world are contagious. We can transform our worlds into ones that support health and justice by each practicing on the small scale the patterns of change that we hope to achieve in our larger systems.

"Emergence is the way complex systems and patterns arise out of a multiplicity of relatively simple interactions," teaches adrienne maree brown, in *Emergent Strategy: Shaping Change, Changing Worlds.* In this way, we can leverage our relatively simple interactions to create complex patterns, systems, and transformations to create healthier possibilities on a large scale.

Central to strengthening our network's connections is building trust among each other. "Many of us have been socialized to understand that constant growth, violent competition, and critical mass are the ways to create change," brown explains. "But emergence shows us that adaptation and evolution depend more upon critical, deep, and authentic connections . . . the quality of connection between the nodes in the patterns. Dare I say love," brown continues. "The strength of our movement is in the strength of our relationships, which could only be measured by their depth."

Brown offers the great migrations of birds as an example:

> They feel a call in their bodies that they must go, and they follow it, responding to each other, each bringing their adaptations. There is an art to flocking: staying separate enough not to crowd each other, aligned enough to maintain a shared direction, and cohesive enough to always move towards each other . . . Each creature is shifting direction, speed, and proximity based on the information of the other creature's bodies. There is a deep trust in this: to lift because the birds around you are lifting, to live based on your collective real-time adaptations. . . . Imagine our movements cultivating this type of trust and depth with each other, having strategic flocking in our playbooks.

When we embrace the reality of our interdependence and build trust and compassion between our many members and connections, there are boundless possibilities in how we can support our collective's transformation to health. And no one person needs to do it all. Instead, each small act of mutual aid and reciprocal care builds communities where, as adrienne maree brown teaches, "we can truly lean on others and they can lean on us."

Reciprocity empowers every one of us to connect and cooperate to share resources, skills, and support to meet each other's needs in decentralized ways, especially when our larger structures of society have yet do so. This care for our collective moves away from the extractive culture and power imbalances of dominance, division, and indifference that's been making us all sick for too long and toward empowering each of us within our own relationships and communities to strengthen our bonds of trust, empathy, and belonging.

These offerings aren't linear transactions where each act must be reciprocated in the same way at the same time to the same person. Instead, we can celebrate our diverse skills and resources to care for the many parts of our collective in a variety of ways, with each seemingly small offering rippling into a larger movement that is greater than the sum of its parts. As Sufi Master Hafiz explained, "Even after all this time, the sun never says to the Earth, 'You owe me.' Look what happens with a love like that! It lights up the whole sky."

We're still waiting for our world's happy endings, where we overcome our harmful dynamics to transform the pieces of our broken systems into something more gorgeous than we've ever known. While we still haven't emerged into a new state of balance, we're learning how to get there.

THE GIFT OF IMPERMANENCE

our world keeps breaking, over and over again.
i have no choice but to believe that a new one is being born.
—KAI CHENG THOM

———

I'M SITTING WITH A GROUP OF WOMEN AND GENDER DIVERSE FOLKS FROM AROUND THE world at a climate gathering on Cortes Island in July of 2025, close to my home on the BC coast, sharing in grief and gratitude for the ninety-six-year-old visionary teacher, social and environmental activist and scholar Joanna Macy, as she lay in hospice, taking her last breaths of this gorgeous world that she fought so hard to protect.

Grief is a compass to our heart, showing us what matters, a gift, if held in gratitude, with its waves reminding us of our deep connection to this world.

Joanna Macy knew how to love. "To be alive in this beautiful, self-organizing universe—to participate in the dance of life with sense to perceive it, lungs that breathe it, organs that draw nourishment from it—is a wonder beyond words," she said. Macy taught us to love beyond the fictional borders of our own bodies, partners, families, and nations, naming her workshops the Work That Reconnects. "We are the Earth," she taught. "When we see the world as self, we fall in love with the world. When we fall in love with someone, we want to be with them, serve them, protect them."

Macy also knew how to grieve. "Remember that the heart that breaks open can hold the whole universe," Macy offered. We can make "good, rich compost out of all that grief," she taught, learning from our losses to enhance our larger, collective knowing.

Her love and grief for our ailing planet fueled her actions to protect it. Macy believed we can emerge from the cancer of late-stage capitalism's "industrial growth society" of inequities, violence, and overextraction—what she called the Great Unraveling—to regenerate and flourish into a "life-sustaining society" of ecological and social balance. She called this collective movement toward health the Great Turning. Not only do we need to stop the ongoing harm and slow the damage of our cancerous dynamics of dominance, division, and indifference, but we must also transform our structures into just and sustainable systems that once again support life.

The Great Turning requires a change in our world view so that we recognize our interdependence with all the parts of our Earth that need our loving attention and care. Inspired by the Tibetan Buddhist oral tradition of the Shambhala Warrior Prophecy, as taught to her by her dear friend, Druga Choegyal Rinpoche, a Tibetan lama exiled to the Tashi Jong community in northern India, Macy shared the emergence of the Kingdom of Shambhala:

> There comes a time when all life on Earth is in danger. In this time, great powers have arisen, barbarian powers. And although they waste their wealth in preparations to annihilate each other, they have much in common. And among the things they have in common, are weapons of unfathomable death and devastation and technologies that lay waste to the world. And it is just in this time when the future of all beings is to hang by the frailest of threads that the Kingdom of Shambhala emerges.
>
> Now you cannot go there because it's not a place. It exists in the hearts and minds of Shambhala warriors. And you can't tell a Shambhala warrior by looking at them because there's no uniforms,

no insignia, no banners to declare what side you're on. No barricades on which you can rest and regroup or stand to threaten the enemy, nor any home turf because always and ever you just have the terrain of the barbarian powers to move across.

Now the time has come that requires great courage of the warriors—moral courage and physical courage—because they are going to go to the very center of the barbarian powers to dismantle their weapons. They are going to go into the pits where the armouries are made and deployed and also go into the corridors of power where the decisions are made and dismantle those weapons too. The Shambhala warriors know they can dismantle these weapons because they are *manomaya* or mind made. That means they are made by the human mind so they can be unmade by the human mind . . . they arise from our choices, our habits, our relationships.

So now is the time the Shambala warriors go into training. They train in the use of two weapons . . . one is compassion, and the other is insight into the radical interdependence of all phenomena. And you need both. One is not enough.

You need compassion because that provides the fuel to where you need to go and to do what you need to do. And what it boils down to is not being afraid of the suffering of our world. And when you're not afraid of the pain, then nothing can stop you. But by itself, that's so hot, that fuel: It can burn you out. So you need the other.

You need the insight into the radical interdependence of all things. And with that you know this is not a battle between the good guys and the bad guys, but that the line between good and evil runs through the landscape of every human heart. And that we are so interwoven in the web of existence that even the smallest act with clear intention has repercussions that we can't begin to see, let alone measure. But that, while essential, is a little cool, a little abstract, so you need the heat of compassion too.[1]

Macy reminded us that it's not the first time radical transformations emerged in our societies. The agricultural and industrial revolutions are only two of many major shifts that changed the structures
and values of how we live. And they are only brief blips within the
long history of humankind. If we were to imagine all of human history as a twenty-four-hour clock, Macy taught, Christopher Colum-
bus didn't reach Turtle Island (North America) until three minutes
before midnight, and the Industrial Revolution began in the last two
minutes. "In the last twenty seconds (that is, since 1950), we have used
up more resources and fuel than in all human history before this,"
Macy explained. And if we were to symbolize the entire history of our
planet on a twenty-four-hour clock, humans only entered the picture
in the last five seconds.

For many of us, it may feel like we've only known this one world,
this industrial growth society, as a viable option for humanity. But if
we zoom out, we can imagine the boundless possibilities in the path
ahead for many alternative ways to live.

We're already in the process of liberating ourselves from the per-
vasive dynamics of harm that we've been marinating in for too long.
"If the world is to be healed through human efforts, I am convinced it
will be ordinary people, people whose love for this life is even greater
than their fear," Macy shared. She invited us to acknowledge and ap-
preciate all the ways we are already turning up to create a new world:

- WHERE and how are you turning up?
- WHAT are you turning away from because you know it causes harm?
- WHAT are you turning toward because it aligns more strongly with
  your values and hopes for our future?

As Macy lay in hospice herself, so many of us gathering on Cortes Island are reading and sharing the teachings of Brazilian educator, Indigenous activist, and former Canada Research Chair in Race,
Inequalities and Global Change Vanessa Machado de Oliveira An-

dreotti, who wrote *Hospicing Modernity*. Modernity, like Macy's "industrial growth society," Andreotti explains, is the cancerous story of the promise of comfort and security from unlimited growth with the denial of our complicity in the historical, structural, and ongoing violence, injustices, and unsustainability required to uphold it.

"'Living better' is commonly promoted in modernity's ladder of social mobility, feeding the perceived needs to constantly aspire to have more than one has and more than one's neighbours," explains Andreotti. "In contrast, the term 'living well' (*buen vivir*) is often understood to be an Andean philosophy that . . . emphasiz[es] the centrality of 'having enough' in order to sustain reciprocal relations between all living beings," she continues. However, *buen vivir* is partly an attempted translation of the Quechua term *sumac kawsay*, she explains, a living practice of both "living well" and "dying well" as part of the same cycle—to prepare for the inevitable rhythms of pain, loss, and change.

Rather than clinging to the dying story of modernity, we can co-evolve to see, feel, relate, desire, and imagine otherwise, teaches Andreotti. And to do so, we must hospice modernity, accepting that its story is expiring, learning from its mistakes—including how we're all entangled within its harms—and then releasing it so we can adopt healthier possibilities. "The end of the world as we know it is not necessarily the end of the world," she explains "We can think about it instead as the end of a harmful habit of being, which has become untenable."

Machado de Oliveira Andreotti offers the popular saying in Brazil: In a flood, it's only when the water reaches people's hips that it becomes possible for them to swim. "We might only be able to learn to swim—that is, to exist differently—once we have no other choice," she explains.

As the water keeps rising, we see that all the ailing parts of this poly-crisis are interconnected and caused by modernity's relationally unethical and ecologically unsustainable structures, Andreotti explains.

Rather than desperately trying to resuscitate a dying model, we can offer it palliative care. Hospicing understands the necessity of enabling a "good" death through which important lessons are processed, she explains. "These lessons are learned through the accomplishments and mistakes of the dying system, so that they can be applied as we witness and help midwife the birth of something different."

In her memoir, *A Body across Two Hemispheres*, Victoria Buitron describes an Ecuadorian holiday where they spend weeks building temporary sculptures of wood, cardboard, and newspaper to create effigies that represent the past year. The men then dress up as widows in borrowed black dresses and parade their creations around until midnight, when they use explosives and gasoline to burn them to ash on the street. "Art created for destruction," Buitron explains. When we watch what we've created turn to dust, we continue the tradition of letting go of our tight grip on the past and accepting the impermanence of reality.

"Awareness that all things pass away is inescapable for anyone who pays attention," wrote poet John Brehm.[2] "Of course, our culture encourages us not to pay attention, to live as if we will live forever, as if we can plunder the Earth unceasingly and without consequence." He continued, quoting Master Dōgen: "What dreamwalkers men become."

While we keep sleepwalking to the edge of the cliff, following our collective to the brink of losing it all—our health, our world, and our humanity—maybe it's the fragility of this moment in time that will save us all. Maybe we need to be threatened with extinction for all our bodies to jolt awake in a loud stop sign to halt our mindless support of the status quo. Because the status quo has been hurting us for ages. Maybe the intensity of our collective distress is finally enough motivation to transform our world into one that sustains life, into one that unites and shares and loves and cares.

As a kid, I always assumed that Earth as I knew it would go on forever, and with so many years ahead of me, it felt like I would, too.

But as I've stopped clinging to these fantasies, I'm free to live with intention and purpose, gushing with awe and gratitude for the miracles of our intricate web of life and the love and belonging that come from connecting to it all.

In my training with Buddhist teacher Jack Kornfield, he shared a lesson from his Thai mentor, Ajahn Chah. "You see this teacup?" asked Chah. "To me, this cup is already broken. Because I know its fate, I can enjoy it fully here and now. But when I put this cup on the shelf and the wind knocks it over, or my elbow brushes it off the table and it falls to the ground and shatters, I say, 'Of course.' When I understand that the glass is already broken, every moment with it is precious."[3] When we accept how fragile it all is, we learn to never take anything for granted.

As poet Mary Oliver asks, "Tell me, what is it you plan to do / with your one wild and precious life?"

IN GRATITUDE

To my Rat Park: my incredible kids, co-parent, Mom, Dad, brother, extended family, chosen family (my lifeboat of joy and support), and my dear love for all of your ongoing care, cheerleading, and patience. I know how lucky I am.

To my agent/therapist/superhero Marilyn Biderman at Transatlantic Agency, who made this all happen with such skill, grace, confidence, and joy: you're my winning lottery ticket and I'm forever in awe of my immense fortune in finding you. To my primary editor, Brad Wilson at HarperCollins Canada, who proves that the strongest among us are those who are the most gentle, connected, and compassionate: thank you for making the journey of publishing a book as warm and cozy as curling up on the couch to read one. Your confidence in this project from the very beginning has been contagious. To my co-editors Francis Bickmore at Canongate and Renee Sedliar at Balance, for your continuous support and enthusiasm throughout the process. To my editor Nicole Langlois, for your patience and tact in helping me find the right dose of asshole and cutting and shaping all those excessive words in my early drafts.

To Ellie Parton, for the warming joy of your friendship, audiobook narration, and ongoing collaboration: I feel so lucky to join our voices. To my dear friend Jackie Duys, for the illustrations, daily love, and holding my hand through the horrors of headshots. To Dr. Randi

George, who spent countless hours with me editing and discussing the manuscript, helping me uncover my unconscious biases and exploring how the concepts of the book apply across different cultures and positions of power and privilege: I can't wait to read your future books and for the world to share in the gifts of your wisdom. To Anya Phillip, who's spent years as a role model championing EDI and anti-oppression work in our mental health programs, for so generously editing my manuscript: Your courage and passion have led to huge waves of growth throughout our entire community. Thank you for starting these essential conversations in our organizations and helping me learn and grow. To Yasmin Hajian, for supporting me in building the strength to show up and hold my privilege and power in healthy ways, and for offering such a soft landing when shame keeps pushing me into hiding. To Sam Fletcher, for making the process a living paradise. To Ali Hall, for all the hours of body doubling, loving therapy, and systems theory geek outs. To Erin Burrell, the best friend and work wife I could ever imagine, for your support, inspiration, genius, and having the actual skills to put my passion into action. To Morgan Rich, for all the joy, nurturing, and love of my chaos. To Norbert Kouri, who literally carried me to the finish line. To my co-conspirator, Rummy Dosanjh, for your infectious optimism and passion to fight for a better world. To Kristie Wightman, for your gorgeous heart and constant support through the process. To Chantal Bourke, for your gooey love and constant cheerleading. I feel so grateful to have been held by this big family of gentle brilliance.

To the teachers who unknowingly showed me other ways to live: bell hooks, who linked self-help with political resistance to our culture of dominance in *Sisters of the Yam* (1993); Toni Morrison, Ocean Vuong, adrienne maree brown, Naomi Klein, and all the writers who've been my steady imaginary friends over the years. To Tara Brach and Jack Kornfield, for embodying the kind of teacher, writer, therapist, and human I aspire to become. To Dr. Dan J. Siegel and Dr. Gabor Maté, who so courageously failed to stay in their doctor lanes. To

Dan, your power to integrate and understand the science and soul of mental health can only be described as genius. To Gabor, who continues to show up every time I need inspiration and mentorship on how to live as a physician who speaks up against injustice: thank you for your generous support with my foreword and for showing me how to be a doctor with integrity. To Trudy Goodman, Kelly S. Thompson, Cooper Lee Bombardier, and Shelley Robertson, who believed in me way before I did.

To my many therapists, patients, participants, and students, for teaching me more than anyone else.

To our gorgeous collective, who constantly inspires me with so many acts of love and care and wonder. I can't wait to witness our happy endings. And to DD, for each gorgeous moment together, and for our future.

NOTES

INTRODUCTION

1. Freud, S., & Breuer, J. (2004). *Studies in hysteria.* (N. Luckhurst, Trans.). Penguin Press.
2. Nesse, R. M. (2019). *Good reasons for bad feelings: Insights from the frontier of evolutionary psychiatry.* Dutton.
3. Adapted from Siegel, R. (2014). *The science of mindfulness: A research-based path to well-being.* The Great Courses.
4. Klein, N. (2023). *Doppelganger: A trip into the mirror world.* Knopf Canada.
5. Linehan, M. (1993). *Cognitive behavioral treatment of borderline personality disorder.* Guilford Press.

ONE: WE'VE EVOLVED TO SURVIVE, AND BE MISERABLE

1. Canadian Mental Health Association. (2021). *Fast facts about mental illness.* Canadian Mental Health Association. https://cmha.ca/brochure/fast-facts-about-mental-illness/
2. Gilbert, P. (2019). *Living like crazy* (2nd revised ed.). Annwyn House.
3. Panksepp J. (2010). Affective neuroscience of the emotional BrainMind: evolutionary perspectives and implications for understanding depression. *Dialogues in Clinical Neuroscience, 12*(4), 533–545.
4. Nesse, R. (2022). Evolutionary psychiatry [Video]. HSTalks. https://hstalks.com/t/4946/evolutionary-psychiatry/?biosci.
5. Owens, R. (2020). *Love and rage: The path of liberation through anger.* North Atlantic Books.
6. Nesse, R. (2019). *Good reasons for bad feelings: Insights from the frontier of evolutionary psychiatry.* Dutton.
7. Rakoff, V. (1966). A long term effect of the concentration camp experience. *Viewpoints, 1,* 17–22.
8. Yehuda, R., & Giller, E. (1994). Comments on the lack of integration between the Holocaust and PTSD literatures. *PTSD Research Quarterly, 5,* 5–7.
9. Yehuda, R., & Lehrner, A. (2018). Intergenerational transmission of trauma effects: Putative role of epigenetic mechanisms. *World Psychiatry, 17*(3), 243–257.
10. Yehuda, R. (2022). How parents' trauma leaves biological traces in children: Adverse experiences can change future generations through epigenetic pathways. *Scientific*

American. https://www.scientificamerican.com/article/how-parents-rsquo-trauma-leaves-biological-traces-in-children/

11. Nesse, R. (2015). Emotional evolution. In D. F. Sieff, *Understanding and healing emotional trauma: Conversations with pioneering clinicians and researchers.* Routledge.

12. Chisholm, J. S. (2015). Live fast, die young: An evolved response to hostile environments? In *Understanding and healing emotional trauma: Conversations with pioneering clinicians and researchers.* Routledge.

13. Yazeed, C. (2023, April 5). *Black women and vulnerability: What Brene Brown got wrong.* Dr. Carey Yazeed. https://drcareyyazeed.com/black-women-and-vulnerability-what-brene-brown-got-wrong/

TWO: SELF-CARE IS COLLECTIVE-CARE

1. Machado, S., Kyriopoulos, I., Orav, E. J., & Papanicolas, I. (2025). Association between wealth and mortality in the United States and Europe. *The New England Journal of Medicine,* 392 (13), 1310–1319.

2. Institute of Medicine and National Research Council. (2013). *U.S. health in international perspective: Shorter lives, poorer health.* The National Academies Press. https://doi.org/10.17226/13497

3. Bezruchka, S., Namekata, T., & Sistrom, M. G. (2008.) Improving economic equality and health: The case of postwar Japan. *American Journal of Public Health,* 98, 589–594.

4. Wilkinson, R. G. (1992). Income distribution and life expectancy. *British Medical Journal,* 18;304(6820), 165–168.

5. Pickett, K. E., & Wilkinson, R. G. (2015). Income inequality and health: A causal review. *Social Science & Medicine,* 128(C), 316–326.

6. Schenkman, S., & Bousquat, A. (2021). From income inequality to social inequity: Impact on health levels in an international efficiency comparison panel. *BMC Public Health,* 21, 688.

7. Wilkinson, R. D., & Pickett, K. (2009). *The spirit level: Why more equal societies almost always do better.* Allen Lane/Penguin Group UK.

8. Schenkman, S., & Bousquat, A. (2021). From income inequality to social inequity: Impact on health levels in an international efficiency comparison panel. *BMC Public Health,* 21, 688.

9. Wilkinson, R. G., & Pickett, K. E. (2024). Why the world cannot afford the rich. *Nature,* Mar;627(8003), 268–270.

10. The Equality Trust. (2023). *Cost of Inequality 2023.* https://media.equality-trust.out.re/uploads/2023/11/ReportCostofInequality-1.pdf.

11. National Geographic Society. (2023, October 25). *Land management declined as Native Americans were displaced.* https://education.nationalgeographic.org/resource.

12. Tutu, D. (2012). *No future without forgiveness.* Ebury Publishing.

13. Stuit, H. (2016). Ubuntu and common humanity in the South African Truth and Reconciliation Commission. In *Ubuntu strategies: Constructing spaces of belonging in contemporary South African culture.* Palgrave Macmillan.

14. Capra, F., & Luisi, P. L. (2014). *The systems view of life: A unifying vision.* Cambridge University Press.

15. Capra, F., & Luisi, P. L. (2014). *The systems view of life: A unifying vision.* Cambridge University Press.

16. Siegel, D. (2022). *Intraconnected: Mwe (me + we) as the integration of self, identity, and belonging.* W. W. Norton.

17. Capra, F., & Luisi, P. L. (2014). *The systems view of life: A unifying vision.* Cambridge University Press.

18. Capra, F., & Luisi, P. L. (2014). *The systems view of life: A unifying vision.* Cambridge University Press.

19. Janis, I. L. (1972). *Victims of groupthink: A psychological study of foreign-policy decisions and fiascoes.* Houghton Mifflin.

20. Livesley, W. J. (2012). Integrated treatment: A conceptual framework for an evidence-based approach to the treatment of personality disorders. *Journal of Personality Disorders,* 26(1), 17–42.

21. Hofmann, S. G., & Hayes, S. C. (2019). The future of intervention science: Process-based therapy. *Clinical Psychological Science,* Jan;7(1), 37–50.

22. Barlow, D. H., Farchione, T. J., Bullis, J. R., Gallagher, M. W., Murray-Latin, H., Sauer-Zavala, S., Bentley, K. H., Thompson-Hollands, J., Conklin, L. R., Boswell, J.F., Ametaj, A., Carl, J. R., Boettcher, H. T., & Cassiello-Robbins, C. (2017, September). The unified protocol for transdiagnostic treatment of emotional disorders compared with diagnosis-specific protocols for anxiety disorders: A randomized clinical trial. *JAMA Psychiatry,* 1;74(9), 875–884.

THREE: A WORLD INFLAMED

1. Cole, S. W. (2013.) Social regulation of human gene expression: Mechanisms and implications for public health. *American Journal of Public Health,* 103 (Suppl 1), S84–92.

2. Cole, S. W. (2014.) Human social genomics. *PLOS Genetics,* 10 (8), e1004601.

3. Li, X., Li, C., Zhang, W. et al. (2023). Inflammation and aging: Signaling pathways and intervention therapies. *Signal Transduction and Targeted Therapy,* 8, 239.

4. Hughes, K., Bellis, M. A., Hardcastle, K. A., Sethi, D., Butchart, A., Mikton, C., Jones, L., & Dunne, M. P. (2017, August). The effect of multiple adverse childhood experiences on health: A systematic review and meta-analysis. *Lancet Public Health,* 2(8):e356-e366.

5. Ontario Agency for Health Protection and Promotion. (2020). Interventions to prevent and mitigate the impact of adverse childhood experiences (ACEs) in Canada: a literature review. Public Health Ontario. Queen's Printer for Ontario.

6. Zhang, F. F., Peng, W., Sweeney, J. A., Jia, Z. Y., & Gong, Q. Y. (2018). Brain structure alterations in depression: Psychoradiological evidence. *CNS Neuroscience & Therapeutics,* 24, 994–1003.

7. Rădulescu, I., Drăgoi, A. M., Trifu, S. C., & Cristea, M. B. (2021, October). Neuroplasticity and depression: Rewiring the brain's networks through pharmacological therapy (review). *Experimental and Therapeutic Medicine,* 22(4), 1131.

8. Nusslock, R., Alloy, L. B., Brody, G. H., & Miller, G. E. (2024). Annual research review: Neuroimmune network model of depression: a developmental perspective. *Journal of Child Psychology and Psychiatry, and Allied Disciplines,* 65(4), 538–567.

9. Peay, H. L., & Austin, J. C. (2011). *How to talk with families about genetics and psychiatric illness.* W. W. Norton & Company.

10. Daniel Siegel first mentioned ABC in an enneagram lecture to describe the counter-

parts to our subcortical threats, referring to agency, bonding, and certainty, in reference to different personality patterns.

11. West, J., & Warner, C. (2019). *Combat and operational stress control.* In Office of the Surgeon General, Fundamentals of military medicine. Borden Institute Publishing.

12. Walter Reed Army Institute of Research. (2020). COVID-19 iCOVER-Med. https://media.defense.gov/2023/Apr/11/2003197390/-1/-1/1/ICOVER-MED -COVID-19-QUICK-GUIDE-WRAIR-V1.PDF.

13. National Council of Certified Dementia Practitioners. *The four R's of dementia care: A guide for caregivers.* https://www.nccdp.org/the-four-rs-of-dementia-care-a-guide-for -caregivers/

14. Nelson-Coffey, S. K., Fritz, M. M., Lyubomirsky, S., & Cole, S. W., (2017). Kindness in the blood: A randomized controlled trial of the gene regulatory impact of prosocial behavior. *Psychoneuroendocrinology*, 81, 8–13.

15. Kitayama, S., Akutsu, S., Uchida, Y., & Cole, S. W. (2016). Work, meaning, and gene regulation: Findings from a Japanese information technology firm. *Psychoneuroendo-crinology*, 72, 175–181.

16. Seeman, T., Merkin, S. S., Goldwater, D., & Cole, S. W. (2020, January). Intergenera-tional mentoring, eudaimonic well-being and gene regulation in older adults: A pilot study. *Psychoneuroendocrinology*, 111:104468.

17. Kitayama, S., Akutsu, S., Uchida, Y., & Cole, S. W. (2016.) Work, meaning, and gene regulation: Findings from a Japanese information technology firm. *Psychoneu-roendocrinology*, 72, 175–181. Fredrickson, B. L., Grewen, K. M., Algoe, S. B., et al. (2015). Psychological well-being and the human conserved transcriptional response to adversity. *PLOS One*, 10 (3), e0121839.

18. Seeman, T., Merkin, S. S., Goldwater, D., & Cole, S. W. (2020, January). Intergenera-tional mentoring, eudaimonic well-being and gene regulation in older adults: A pilot study. *Psychoneuroendocrinology*. 111:104468.

19. Maynard, R., & Betasomasake Simpson, L. (2022). *Rehearsals for Living.* Penguin Random House: Vintage Canada.

20. Kelly, M. (2014). Living enterprises as a foundation of a generative economy. In F. Capra & P. L. Luisi, *The systems view of life: A unifying vision.* Cambridge University Press.

21. www.democracycollaborative.org.

22. Capra, F., & Luisi, P. L. (2014). *The systems view of life: A unifying vision.* Cambridge University Press.

23. Capra, F., & Luisi, P. L. (2014). *The systems view of life: A unifying vision.* Cambridge University Press.

FOUR: WE ARE OUR HISTORY

1. Menakem, R. (2017). *My grandmother's hands.* Central Recovery Press.

2. Macy, J. (2015, March 17). Joanna Macy talks about the Kingdom of Shambhala. Mountains and Rivers Order. https://mountainsangha.org/joanna-macy-talks-about -the-kingdom-of-shambhala/.

3. For more information on nonviolent communication, see *Nonviolent communication: A language of life: Life-changing tools for healthy relationships* (2015) by Marshall Rosenberg and Deepak Chopra.

4. This concept is referred to as idealization and devaluation in object relations therapy, all or nothing or black and white thinking in cognitive therapy, and the I hate you; don't leave me of frenemies and clashing lovers.

5. Duran, E. (2019). *Trauma-informed counseling Indigenous communities* (2nd ed). Teachers College Press.

6. Ross, R. (2002). *Exploring criminal justice and the Aboriginal healing paradigm.* Presented to Association for the Treatment of Sexual Abusers: 21st Annual Research and Treatment Conference, Montreal, Quebec. Referenced in Linklater, R. (2014). *Decolonizing trauma work: Indigenous stories and strategies.* Fernwood Publishing.

7. Couture, J. E. (2005). *Approaching Aboriginal assessment issues.* Unpublished manuscript. Referenced in Linklater, R. (2014). *Decolonizing trauma work: Indigenous stories and strategies.* Fernwood Publishing.

8. Society for the Study of Myth and Tradition. (2002). Parabola: War, 27, 4. Daimon.

9. Torrelli, C. (2020). Those who suffered the most were the people: Composer of explosive violence in Cambodia, and the power of music to heal. *Action on Armed Violence.*

10. Brave Heart, M. Y. H. (1998). The return to the sacred path: Healing the historical trauma and historical unresolved grief response among the Lakota through a psychoeducational group intervention. *Smith College Studies of Social Work,* 68, 3, 287–305. Linklater, R. (2014). *Decolonizing trauma work: Indigenous stories and strategies.* Fernwood Publishing.

11. Omar, D. (1995). *Promotion of National Unity and Reconciliation Act*, No 34.

12. Tutu, D. (2012). *No future without forgiveness.* Ebury Publishing.

13. Rhydderch, T. (2022). An instrument in state-building: reconsidering the role of South Africa's Truth and Reconciliation Commission. *FLUX International Relations Review, 12(1).*

14. Ministry of Justice and Constitutional Development. (2024). *The Truth and Reconciliation Commission.* Justice.gov.za.

15. Rhydderch, T. (2022). An instrument in state-building: reconsidering the role of South Africa's Truth and Reconciliation Commission. *FLUX International Relations Review, 12(1).*

16. Lee, S. E., & Dahinten, V. S. (2021, November). Psychological safety as a mediator of the relationship between inclusive leadership and nurse voice behaviors and error reporting. *Journal of Nursing Scholarship,* 53(6), 737–745.

17. Morrow, K. J., Gustavson, A. M., & Jones, J. (2016). Speaking up behaviours (safety voices) of healthcare workers: A metasynthesis of qualitative research studies. *International Journal of Nursing Studies,* 64, 42–51. Lee, S. E., & Dahinten, V. S. (2021, November). Psychological safety as a mediator of the relationship between inclusive leadership and nurse voice behaviors and error reporting. *Journal of Nursing Scholarship,* 53(6), 737–745.

FIVE: HOW TO BE AN ANTI-ASSHOLE

1. As part of the Gesturing toward Decolonial Futures Collective, University of Victoria's Vanessa Machado de Oliveira Andreotti, the former Canada Research Chair in Race, Inequalities and Global Change, also uses the term *Anti-asshole* in an Anti-assholism memo to help us unlearn our harmful unconscious colonial wiring, especially of hyper-individualism, hyper-consumerism and narcissism.

2. Diangelo, R. (2018). *White fragility: Why it's so hard for white people to talk about racism.* Beacon Press.

3. McCown, D., Reibel, D. K., & Micozzi, M. S. (2010). Teaching mindfulness: a practical guide for clinicians and educators. *College of Health Sciences Faculty Books.*

4. This exercise is commonly attributed to Jon Kabat-Zinn, although it is based on Vipassana Buddhism's equanimity practices.

5. Gillespie, C. F. et al. (2020). Unipolar depression. In Rosenberg's M*olecular and genetic basis of neurologic and psychiatric disease* (6th ed., 2nd vol.). Elsevier Academic Press.

6. Hanh, T. N. (2012). *The pocket Thich Nhat Hanh.* Shambhala.

7. Mauss, I. B., Tamir, M., Anderson, C. L., & Savino, N. S. (2011, August). Can seeking happiness make people unhappy? Paradoxical effects of valuing happiness. *Emotion,* 11(4), 807–815.

8. Schooler, J. W., Ariely, D., & Loewenstein, G. (2003). The pursuit and assessment of happiness may be self-defeating. In I. Brocas & J. D. Carrillo (Eds.), *The psychology of economic decisions: Rationality and well-being.* Oxford University Press.

9. Hook, B. (2000). *All about love: new visions.* William Morrow.

10. MacBeth, A., & Gumley, A. (2012). Exploring compassion: A meta-analysis of the association between self-compassion and psychopathology. *Clinical Psychology Review,* 32(6), 545–552.

11. Leary, M. R., Tate, E. B., Adams, C. E., Batts Allen, A., & Hancook, J. (2007). Self-compassion and reactions to unpleasant self-relevant events: The implications of treating oneself kindly. *Journal of Personality and Social Psychology,* 92(5), 887.

12. Neff, K. D., & Costigan, A. P. (2014). Self-compassion, wellbeing, and happiness. *Psychologie in Osterreich,* 114–117.

13. Baumeister, R. F., Campbell, J. D., Krueger, J. I., & Vohs, K. D. (2003). Does high self-esteem cause better performance, interpersonal success, or healthier lifestyles? *Psychological Science in the Public Interest,* 4 (1), 1–44.

14. Neff, K. D., & Costigan, A. P. (2014). Self-compassion, wellbeing, and happiness. *Psychologie in Osterreich,* 114–117.

15. Seligman, M. E. (1995). *The optimistic child.* Houghton Mifflin.

16. Neff, K. (2003). Self-compassion: An alternative conceptualization of a healthy attitude toward oneself. *Self and Identity,* 2, 85–101.

17. Aberson, C. L., Healy, M., & Romero, V. (2000). Ingroup bias and self-esteem: A meta-analysis. *Personality & Social Psychology Review,* 4, 157–173.

18. Brown, B. (2008). *I thought it was just me (but it isn't): Making the journey from "What will people think?" to "I am enough."* Gotham Books.

19. This exercise is one of the self-compassion practices on Dr. Neff's website, self-compassion.org/exercise-2-self-compassion-break.

20. Klimecki, O., Singer, T. (2011). Empathic distress fatigue rather than compassion fatigue? Integrating findings from empathy research in psychology and social neuroscience. In B. Oakley, A. Knafo, G. Madhavan, et al. (Eds), *Pathological altruism.* Oxford University Press.

21. Penagos-Corzo, J. C., Cosio van-Hasselt, M., Escobar, D., Vázquez-Roque, R. A., & Flores, G. (2022, October) Mirror neurons and empathy-related regions in psychopathy: Systematic review, meta-analysis, and a working model. *Social Neuroscience,* 17(5), 462–479.

22. Singer, T., Klimecki, O. M. (2014). Empathy and compassion. *Current Biology*, 24, R875–R878.

23. Lamm, C., et al. (2007). The neural substrate of human empathy: Effects of perspective-taking and cognitive appraisal. *Journal of Cognitive Neuroscience*, 19, 42–58.

24. Dowling, T. (2018, July). Compassion does not fatigue! *Canadian Veterinary Journal*, 59(7), 749–750.

25. Leiberg, S., et al. (2011). Short-term compassion training increases prosocial behavior in a newly developed prosocial game. *PLOS One*, 6:e17798.

26. Weng, H. Y., et al. (2013). Compassion training alters altruism and neural responses to suffering. *Psychological Science*, 24, 1171–1180.

27. Dalai Lama. (2001). *An open heart*. Little, Brown & Company.

28. Dalai Lama. (2001). *An open heart*. Little, Brown & Company.

29. Hanh, T. N. (2012). *The pocket Thich Nhat Hanh*. Shambhala.

SIX: DE-HIJACKING OUR BRAINS

1. Gunaratana, H. (2002). *Mindfulness in plain English*. Wisdom Publications.

2. Ready, R. E., Carvalho, J. O., & Åkerstedt, A. M. (2012). Evaluative organization of the self-concept in younger, midlife, and older adults. *Research on Aging*, 34(1), 56–79.

3. Shell, S. (2016). Why buildings for autistic people are better for everyone. *Semantic Scholar*, 251436122.

4. Robbins, M. (Host) (2023, October 12). Conquer overwhelm: Your ultimate guide to inner peace with the amazing Dr. Thema Bryant (No. 110) [Audio Podcast Episode]. In *The Mel Robbins Podcast*. SiriusXM Podcasts. https://podcasts.apple.com/us/podcast/conquer-overwhelm-your-ultimate-guide-to-inner-peace/id1646101002?i=1000631041974

5. Jones, S. G., Doxsee, C., & Harrington, N. (2020) *The escalating terrorism problem in the United States*. CSIS Brief. https://www.csis.org/analysis/escalating-terrorism-problem-united-states

SEVEN: GETTING OUT OF OUR HEADS

1. Menakem, M. (2017). *My grandmother's hands: Racialized trauma and the pathway to mending our hearts and bodies*. Central Recovery Press.

2. Jones, K., and Okun, T. (2001). *Dismantling racism: A workbook for social change groups*. ChangeWork. www.dismantlingracism.org.

3. Chou, T., et al. (2023). The default mode network and rumination in individuals at risk for depression. *Social Cognitive and Affective Neuroscience*, 18, 1.

4. Coutinho, J. F., et al. (2016). Default mode network dissociation in depressive and anxiety states. *Brain Imaging and Behavior*, 10(1), 147–57.

5. Cayoun, B. (2015). *Mindfulness-integrated CBT for well-being and personal growth: Four steps to enhance inner calm, self-confidence and relationships*. Wiley-Blackwell.

6. Leonard, J. (1970, November 13). Books of the Times. *The New York Times*.

7. Mehta, N. (2011). Mind-body dualism: A critique from a health perspective. *Mens Sana Monographs*, 9(1), 202–209.

8. Mehta, N. (2011). Mind-body dualism: A critique from a health perspective. *Mens Sana Monographs*, 9(1), 202–209.

9. Zhang, Li. (2020). *Anxious China: Inner revolution and politics of psychotherapy*. University of California Press.

10. Barlow, D. H., Farchione, T. J., Bullis, J. R., Gallagher, M. W., Murray-Latin, H., Sauer-Zavala, S., Bentley, K. H., Thompson-Hollands, J., Conklin, L. R., Boswell, J. F., Ametaj, A., Carl, J. R., Boettcher, H. T., & Cassiello-Robbins, C. (2017, September). The unified protocol for transdiagnostic treatment of emotional disorders compared with diagnosis-specific protocols for anxiety disorders: A randomized clinical trial. *JAMA Psychiatry*, 1, 74(9), 875–884.

11. Lane, R. E., et al. (2015). Memory reconsolidation, emotional arousal and the process of change in psychotherapy: New insights from brain science. *Behavioral and Brain Sciences*, 38, e1.

12. Panksepp, J. (2010). Affective neuroscience of the emotional BrainMind: Evolutionary perspectives and implications for understanding depression. *Dialogues in Clinical Neuroscience*, 12(4), 533–545.

13. Greenberg, L. S. (2010). *Emotion-focused therapy: Theory and practice*. APA Press.

14. Lane, R. E., et al. (2015). Memory reconsolidation, emotional arousal and the process of change in psychotherapy: New insights from brain science. *Behavioral and Brain Sciences*, 38, e1.

15. Lane, R. E., et al. (2015). Memory reconsolidation, emotional arousal and the process of change in psychotherapy: New insights from brain science. *Behavioral and Brain Sciences*, 38, e1.

16. Panksepp, J. (2010). Affective neuroscience of the emotional BrainMind: evolutionary perspectives and implications for understanding depression. *Dialogues in Clinical Neuroscience*, 12(4), 533–545.

EIGHT: DON'T BELIEVE EVERYTHING YOU THINK

1. Segal, Z. V., Williams, J. M. G., & Teasdale, J. D. (2013). *Mindfulness-based cognitive therapy for depression* (2nd ed.). The Guilford Press.

2. Segal, Z. V., Williams, J. M. G., & Teasdale, J. D. (2013). *Mindfulness-based cognitive therapy for depression* (2nd ed.). The Guilford Press.

3. Aldao, A., Nolen-Hoeksema, S., & Schweizer, S. (2010). Emotion-regulation strategies across psychopathology: A meta-analytic review. *Clinical Psychology Review*, 30(2), 217–237.

4. Zappas, M., Becker, K., & Walton-Moss, B. (2020). Postpartum anxiety. *The Journal for Nurse Practitioners*, 17, 10, 1016.

5. Fairbrother, N., Collardeau, F., Woody, S., Wolfe, D., & Fawcett, J. (2022). Postpartum thoughts of infant-related harm and obsessive-compulsive disorder: Relation to maternal physical aggression toward the infant. *The Journal of Clinical Psychiatry*, 83(2), 21m14006.

6. Wenzlaff, R., & Wegner, D. (2000). Thought suppression. *Annual Review of Psychology*, 51(1), 59–91.

7. Zhang, Li. (2020). *Anxious China: Inner revolution and politics of psychotherapy*. University of California Press.

8. Solnit, R. (2016). *Hope in the Dark: Untold histories, wild possibilities*. Haymarket Books.

NINE: TAKING BACK THE REINS

1. Richards, D. A., et al. (2016). Cost and outcome of behavioural activation versus cognitive behavioural therapy for depression (COBRA): A randomised, controlled, non-inferiority trial. *Lancet*, 388(10047), 871–880.
2. Driessen, E., et al. (2022). Efficacy and moderators of cognitive therapy versus behavioural activation for adults with depression: Study protocol of a systematic review and meta-analysis of individual participant data. *BJPsych Open*, 10, 8(5), e154.
3. Miralles, F., & Garcia, H. (2017). *Ikigai: The Japanese secret to a long and happy life.* Penguin Life.
4. Adapted from Harris, R. (2009). *ACT made simple: A quick-start guide to ACT basics and beyond.* New Harbinger Publications.
5. Harris, R. (2009). *ACT made simple: A quick-start guide to ACT basics and beyond.* New Harbinger Publications.
6. Scott, H. K., Jain, A., & Cogburn, M. (2023). *Behavior modification.* StatPearls Publishing.

TEN: STAYING IN CONNECTION

1. Mauboules, C. (2020, October 7). *Homelessness & supportive housing strategy.* City of Vancouver Report. https://council.vancouver.ca/20201007/documents/pspc1 presentation.pdf
2. Alexander, B., et al. (1981). Effect of early and later colony housing on oral ingestion of morphine in rats. *Pharmacology Biochemistry and Behavior*, 15, 571–576.
3. Canadian Association of Mental Health. (2020, July). Mental health in Canada: Covid-19 and beyond: CAMH policy advice. https://www.camh.ca/-/media/files/pdfs ---public-policy-submissions/covid-and-mh-policy-paper-pdf.pdf
4. Holt-Lunstad, J., Smith, T. B., & Layton, J. B. (2010, July 27). Social relationships and mortality risk: A meta-analytic review. *PLOS Medicine*, 7(7):e1000316.
5. Smith, T. B., et al. (2021, May 18). Effects of psychosocial support interventions on survival in inpatient and outpatient healthcare settings: A meta-analysis of 106 randomized controlled trials. *PLOS Medicine*, 18(5):e1003595.
6. Uvnas-Moberg, K., & Petersson, M. (2005). Oxytocin, ein Vermittler von Antistress, Wohlbefinden, sozialer Interaktion, Wachstum und Heilung [Oxytocin, a mediator of anti-stress, well-being, social interaction, growth and healing]. *Zeitschrift für Psychosomatische Medizin und Psychotherapie*, 51(1), 57–80.
7. Sandstrom, G. M., & Dunn, E. W. (2014). Social interactions and well-being: The surprising power of weak ties. *Personality and Social Psychology Bulletin*, 40(7), 910–922.
8. Sandstrom, G. M., & Dunn, E. W. (2014). Is efficiency overrated?: Minimal social interactions lead to belonging and positive affect. *Social Psychological and Personality Science*, 5(4), 437–442.
9. Ascigil, E., Gunaydin, G., Selcuk, E., Sandstrom, G. M., & Aydin, E. (2023). Minimal social interactions and life satisfaction: The role of greeting, thanking, and conversing. *Social Psychological and Personality Science*, 16, 2, 202–213.
10. Dunn, E. W., Biesanz, J. C., Human, L. J., & Finn, S. (2007). Misunderstanding the affective consequences of everyday social interactions: The hidden benefits of putting one's best face forward. *Journal of Personality and Social Psychology*, 92(6), 990–1005.

11. Sandstrom, G. & Boothby, E. J. (2020). Why do people avoid talking to strangers? A mini meta-analysis of predicted fears and actual experiences talking to a stranger. *Self and Identity*, 20 (1), 47–71.

12. Jetten, J., Branscombe, N. R., Haslam, S. A., Haslam, C., Cruwys, T., Jones, J. M., et al. (2015). Having a lot of a good thing: Multiple important group memberships as a source of self-esteem. *PLOS One*, 10(5), e0124609.

13. Sandstrom, G., et al. (2022). Talking to strangers: A week-long intervention reduces psychological barriers to social connection. *Journal of Experimental Social Psychology*, 102, 104356.

14. McKay, K. M., Imel, Z. E., & Wampold, B. E. (2006). Psychiatrist effects in the psychopharmacological treatment of depression. *Journal of Affective Disorders, 92*(2–3), 287–290.

15. Weissman, M. M. (2006). A brief history of interpersonal psychotherapy. *Psychiatric Annals*, 36, 553–557.

16. Weissman, M. M. (2006). A brief history of interpersonal psychotherapy. *Psychiatric Annals*, 36, 553–557.

17. Markowitz, J. C., & Weissman, M. M. (2012, March–April). Interpersonal psychotherapy: Past, present and future. *Clinical Psychology & Psychotherapy*, 19(2), 99–105.

18. Weissman, M., et al. (2017). *The guide to interpersonal psychotherapy: Updated and expanded edition*. Oxford Press.

19. Page, C., & Woodland, E. *Healing justice lineages: Dreaming at the crossroads of liberation, collective care, and safety*. North Atlantic Books.

20. Fisher, J. (2017). *Healing the fragmented selves of trauma survivors*. Routledge.

21. Kaba, M., & Hayes, K. (2023). How much discomfort is the whole world worth? Movement building requires a culture of listening—not mastery of the right language. *Boston Review*. https://www.bostonreview.net/articles/how-much-discomfort-is-the-whole-world-worth/.

22. UN Women. (2025). *Women's rights in review 30 years after Beijing*. United Nations Entity for Gender Equality and the Empowerment of Women (UN Women).

23. Le Bon, G. (1895). *The crowd*. Dover Publications.

24. Baldoni, J., Plank, L., Heath, J. (Hosts). (2021, July 26). Alok Vaid-Menon: The urgent need for compassion. [Audio Podcast Episode]. In *The Man Enough Podcast*. Wayfarer Studios LLC. https://podcasts.apple.com/us/podcast/alok-vaid-menon-the-urgent-need-for-compassion/id1571480224?i=1000530016080

25. I can be reached on my website at www.joannacheek.ca.

EPILOGUE: THE GIFT OF IMPERMANENCE

1. Macy, J. "The Kingdom of Shambhala" (Spirit Rock Meditation Center, 2014). Used with permission from Spirit Rock Meditation Center. (c) 2014/2025 Spirit Rock.

2. Brehm, J. (2017). *The poetry of impermanence, mindfulness, and joy*. Wisdom Publications.

3. Epstein, M. (2013). *Thoughts without a thinker: Psychotherapy from a Buddhist perspective*. Basic Books.

INDEX